# Fresh Food Matters

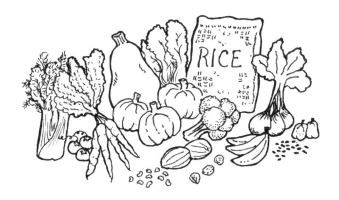

Suzanne Landry
*The Fresh Food Chef*

To my husband, George

# Contents

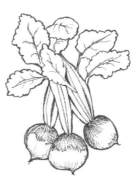

"Good health is our greatest wealth."

# The Birth of My Passion

*"Without good health nothing else in life matters."*
That was one of the many truths my dad taught me when I was growing up. His seventeen years of recurring cancer taught him the value of good health. He died at the young age of forty-seven years. Soon after, I began a journey of my own healing. My dad's death at such young age, my own health challenges, and my children's chronic health problems were the catalysts to my journey. It's been fascinating to explore the connection between food and healing, and thirty years later, I'm still captivated by it.

When I was twenty-eight years old, I suffered from low energy, chronic back problems, digestive disorders, and painful ovarian cysts. My doctor recommended surgery to remove my ovary because of a lemon-sized cyst. At the same time, over an eighteen-month period, my five-year-old son had more than ten episodes of ear infections followed by several bouts of bronchitis. The "cure" offered was traditional antibiotics. Five pediatricians prescribed more than fourteen different antibiotics. At the same time, my eighteen-month old son was suffering from an irritating eczema that began when he was only six months old. The only "remedy" prescribed was hydrocortisone cream. I felt helpless, but unwilling to just treat the symptoms. I kept asking, "What's the cause?" My helplessness turned into stubborn determination as I searched for answers.

Even as a child I felt there was a cause for every effect and that nothing ever "just happened." I knew in my deepest self that there were reasons for everything. This deep searching for truth led me on many paths of study. I came to understand and believe that healing has to be holistic because it addresses the mind and body. True wellness includes both.

We, like most Americans, ate for pleasure and were totally unaware of the tremendous influence our food had on our energy levels, our sleep, our health and our overall sense of well-being. I had subscribed to the Standard American Diet (S.A.D.) which is excessively high in protein, salt and saturated fats, and dangerously low in fiber and complex carbohydrates. The S.A.D. diet is truly sad, and I wanted alternatives. My leisure time became study time. I read everything related to health and nutrition, and I implemented dietary changes that changed our lives. Our transition was slow and steady so these gradual changes were easily incorporated into our daily eating habits. Slow and steady progress is what I still recommend for my students today.

The first change to our diet was to reduce red meat and white sugar. Immediately I felt more energetic, especially in the mornings. I became less irritable and more patient. My family started appreciating the natural taste of fresh vegetables and whole grains. Since I had become bored cooking the S.A.D. diet for my family, I began experimenting with new foods, flavors and textures. Cooking immediately became an exciting and creative adventure. My boys joined me in chopping vegetables, making homemade breads and cookies. They began to feel a part of this new adventure.

*The best news was that with every positive step we made, more of our symptoms disappeared.*

After a few weeks, the eczema and ear infections that plagued my sons were gone, and after several months, my cysts disappeared! It seemed like a miracle then and it still does today.

Good health is within your reach. The road to good health is a joyous journey of learning. Our bodies gently teach us each step of the way. We need only to listen and learn. Our bodies tell us what makes us feel good, what gives us energy and what drains our energy. While it's not always easy to listen and respect these messages, every time we do, we enjoy a greater sense of awareness, self-love and vitality. My journey of good health has been the most important, interesting, rewarding, and yes, sometimes challenging journey in my life. And every step has been worth the effort. "Know thyself" echoes in my mind.

My efforts and commitment have rewarded us. For more than thirty years my family and I have been in good health. None of us have needed medication of any kind—not even aspirin. Even simple colds are very rare, as are most other commonly accepted ailments and doctor visits are seldom needed. Most importantly, we have an abundance of energy and good health.

My dad was right—good health is very important and without it nothing else matters very much. This fundamental belief guides my work as a health counselor, educator and speaker. Since 1987 I have been sharing my love of cooking healthy, delicious foods through classes, articles, newsletters, my website, television programs and now through this book. Whether you are just starting your journey, or looking for fresh ideas and innovative recipes, I hope you find the inspiration you are seeking within these pages.

To your health!

Suzanne

# Chapter 1

## You Are What You Eat

Food is not only sustenance, it is one of the primary sensual pleasures of life. What we eat also has far more influence upon our health than any other single factor in our lives. I have no doubt that health is directly related to diet. Food helps to fuel our body and build new cells, which in turn become tissue, then organ systems and then you! Scientists say our bodies renew themselves every seven years and our brain renews itself every ten years. We are constantly replacing old cells with new ones. So we always have the opportunity to change the quality of our blood to create potential disease or vibrant health and the opportunity to slow down the aging process.

### Are your food choices healthy or a health hazard?

Good health isn't something you get on a visit to the doctor's office or when you buy health insurance. It starts when you purchase healthier fresh food, commit to regular exercise, and choose healthier lifestyle habits.

Our modern diet of overly-processed, refined, and de-vitalized foods, further polluted with chemical additives, is far removed from our natural ancestral diet. Nutritional recommendations today remind us to increase our fiber, lower our refined carbohydrates and restrict foods high in trans-fats. You don't have to be a compulsive label reader if you eat fresh foods. Vegetables, fruits, whole grains, beans, free-range meats, organic dairy, or other real, fresh foods don't have ingredient labels. You find these foods along the periphery of a grocery store; so start there. Just shopping the periphery will help you make healthier choices.

Over the years, I have been asked, "Well, what about my grandparents, they ate just about anything and they lived into their 90s?" My question to those who ask is always, "What was the environment like when your grandparents were born? How much pollution was in the air, water and food then?" Many of our grandparents were raised on food grown in their own backyards. Their own chickens gave them fresh eggs and they drank milk from the local farm, often still warm from the cow! For the first 50 years of our grandparents' lives, they built their *constitutions* with hearty wholesome food. If we look closer, we see that processed refined foods, pesticides and herbicides have only been around since post WWII. Sadly, each new generation is raised on more processed food and exposed to more pollution in the environment than ever before.

## Modern Farming—Better?

In 1935, there were 39 agricultural chemicals (mostly fertilizers) in use. Today there are over 20,000 pesticides registered with the Environmental Protection Agency (EPA) with a total application of over one billion tons per year. According to the EPA, 160 of these are synthetic pesticides that are considered possible carcinogens (cancer causing). In 1939, the pesticide DDT was released and was considered safe at that time, but now banned because of the possible link between DDT and birth defects.

The term "pesticides" used here includes: herbicides, fungicides, insecticides and pesticides. A 2004 study by the Center for Disease Control (CDC) found 100% of subjects studied showed pesticide residue in their blood and urine. Perhaps this is because only an estimated 0.1% of pesticides applied reach their target bugs.

> *Of the 80,000 chemicals in commercial use in the U.S., only about 200 are assessed and approved as safe.*

The rest are on a GRAS list (Generally Regarded As Safe). GRAS means initial studies showed no adverse affects. The chemical is then cautiously approved with a "let's wait and see" approach. Yes, we are all "wait and see" guinea pigs for the pharmaceutical and chemical industries. Environmental experts say we are exposed to over 65,000 chemicals in our environment, water, and food every year. Conventionally-grown produce exposes us to an average of more than 50 different pesticide and herbicide residues still on our food. Peanuts and raisins, for example, can contain traces of more than 80 different chemicals.

Although levels of toxic exposure to farm workers is regulated by the government, studies have shown that families who live on farms have a much greater chance of getting cancer than the general population in America! Usually, there is little or no enforcement of these regulations until it is too late and the workers have already developed health problems.

Organic farming methods are safer for farm workers, rural residents, and consumers, and are a way you can avoid all of these chemicals. More about organic farming later.

## Processed Foods

If spraying pesticides isn't enough, we are next confronted by modern food processing. The number of chemical additives and preservatives used in prepared foods is staggering. Although the amounts are regulated to sub-toxic levels, they don't take into account the accumulated amounts, or the interaction of chemicals with each other. Sadly, most chemical product safety testing does not address these issues. It is not required! It's no wonder the typical American consumes in his/her daily diet more than a hundred different chemical additives. In fact, the current food safety standards set by the FDA are intended for *adults only*. Safe levels for children have never been established! The EPA reports that children are exposed to five times more environmental toxins than adults. The effect on children is much greater than on adults because of their body size and growth rate.

## Depleted Soil = Depleted Food

Large scale farming removes four inches of top soil, stripping vital nutrients (more than 45), micro-organisms, worms and soil culture. Synthetic fertilizers that are then used replace only three major nutrients. The result is depleted soil.

Chemical fertilizers consist of three primary nutrients: nitrogen (N), phosphorus (P), and potassium (K). These three are enough to produce *healthy looking crops*, but lack the other essential micro-nutrients that our bodies and plants need. Lack of proper nutrients results in weaker plants that are more vulnerable to pests and disease, necessitating *more* pesticides and herbicides. Some herbicides actually function by preventing the uptake of key micronutrients, further reducing the nutritional value of our foods.

High crop yields forced through the use of chemical fertilizers often result in nutritionally degraded food. For example, wheat at the turn of the century contained 40% protein. Today protein content falls between 8-12%.

> *Our modern diet of refined food leaves our bodies with a continual yearning, a hunger that no amount of food seems to satisfy. We will eat greater quantities of food when quality in the food is lacking.*

# Frankenfoods

Unlike traditional methods, genetic engineering creates new life forms that would never occur in nature. These, then, create new and unpredictable health and environmental risks. Genes from bacteria, viruses, plants, animals—*even humans*—have already been inserted into common food crops, like corn, soy, canola, and alfalfa, to create *Frankenfoods*.

Genetically Modified Organism (GMO) foods or Genetically Engineered (GE) foods have been in our food supply for many years. Over 14 categories of food have been approved for human consumption. Most recently, alfalfa, sugar beets, and farm-raised salmon have joined the list. Ninety percent of our soy, corn, canola and cotton crops are grown from GMO seeds! In 1997 more than 3.7 million acres were used to grow these crops and today it has jumped to 100 million acres!

Virtually all of us have eaten GMO foods or foods that contain ingredients grown from GMO seeds. Yet, 70% of Americans thought that they have never eaten GMO foods. Over 85% of people polled were against consuming GMO foods and outraged to learn that labeling, as such, is not required.

## Who's Behind All This?

Monsanto has spent over eight billion dollars buying up seed companies and has over 11,000 patents pertinent to seeds, pesticides and agriculture. They patent a gene and insert it into the DNA of another variety, or in some cases, another species. If that variety, once planted, cross pollinates with a non-GMO variety, it results in a new variety. Monsanto can then claim that they own the new variety. Here are just a few of the unique genetically modified genes they are using in their GMO crops:

➢ **Suicide gene**: This gene makes a seed sterile after its first harvest, forcing farmers to purchase new seed each year from . . . guess who? Called a terminator gene, there are 12 patents on it. Co-owner of this terminator patent is the US government!

➢ **Germination:** They have proprietary chemicals to make their GMO seeds germinate, locking the farmer into more dependence on this chemical giant.

➢ **Glyphosate herbicide**: This is the active ingredient in **Roundup Ready™,** another Monsanto product. GMO vegetable crops are genetically engineered to survive direct application of **Roundup.** Farmers planting GMO sugar beets are told they *may apply the herbicide up to five times per year,* contaminating both soil and our underground springs!

• **Monsanto's BT corn™** (bacterium Bacillus Thuringiensis) is registered as an insecticide because every cell of the corn has been engineered to produce the BT toxin. The BT bacteria are common bacteria found in the soil and are toxic to corn worms. Remember this is 90% of our corn crop!

• Monsanto was the originator of **DDT ™** , **Agent Orange™** and **Weed Killer 24D™** all now considered to be carcinogenic and may cause birth defects.

Human growth hormones have been crossed with salmon to produce bigger fish. Fish genes have been crossed with tomatoes to give us a tomato that withstands colder temperatures. The list goes on. It is not just in our food. Insects, poultry, trees, and livestock are other areas of GMO interest, which should be our concern as well.

## What's the Motivation?

According to the World Health Organization (WHO), genetically modified food is produced to be more resistant to plant diseases, insects, viruses, pesticides and herbicides. The ultimate goal is for farmers to have a greater food yield and make food cheaper and/or to last longer presumably for the export market. However, the European Union, as of this writing, has refused U.S. imports of any food that has been genetically modified.

The impact of GMO food on the environment is simple and frightening. Its effects cannot be reversed. Unlike other types of pollution (such as chemicals and waste), genetic coding has the potential to spread through pollination in all the ways that life already does. Further, we don't know if the genetic material will combine with human genetic material, causing protein mutation. We just don't know enough about the long term effects these crops will have on all life. Instead, we should be looking for solutions that are based on ecological and biological principles that have fewer environmental costs. Dare we risk future crops and our future generations on a new technology that has not proven to be safe?

By 2003 the U.S. sold millions of pounds of GMO corn to Mexico for less than the cost of growing their own seeds because it was subsidized by American tax payers. GMO corn seeds are sterile and will not produce a fertile seed for another generation. When this seed cross-pollinates with the existing crops, it sterilizes them. Once GMO corn began to cross pollinate with native corn varieties (over 400), Mexico banned all GMO corn planting. But the damage has been done; the GMO pollen is now within the species of corn and will continue to spread.

There is so much more to learn about GMO. Please become informed. Reading labels will not tell you if it contains GMO ingredients, so know the foods that most likely have been genetically modified and look for those ingredients on the label. The following is a short list of foods we know presently that have been genetically modified:

- More than 90% of corn, soy, cotton and canola seeds are genetically engineered. All the by-products from these foods are affected. Watch for high fructose corn syrup, corn solids, corn syrup, glucose syrup, etc. as just some of the by-products of GMO corn. When you buy fresh corn this year, ask the grower if it is GMO free. If it is BT corn, avoid it.
- Buying organic soy products will help you avoid GMO. Read your labels. Most of the breakfast protein bars on the market contain some soy ingredient—potentially from GMO soy.
- GMO modified alfalfa, white sugar beets, and farm-raised salmon have been introduced this year.

- Small amounts of summer squash and papaya are also GMO.

If you want to avoid GMO foods, buy organic. Organic standards do not allow seeds that have been genetically modified to be used. The origin of fresh produce may be indicated on the sticker:

SKU labels (on the produce sticker) will give you a hint as to how food was grown:

- If it is a 4-digit number, the food is conventionally produced.
- If it is a 5-digit number beginning with an 8, it is GMO. However, do not trust that GMO foods will be identified as such, because labeling is optional.
- If it is a 5-digit number beginning with a 9, it is organic.

## What Can We Do About GMO Foods?

1. **Support legislation** that will enforce strict industry standards for the labeling of GMO.
2. **Buy organic.** The most powerful voice you can have is the vote that you make each and every time you shop. With every dollar you spend to buy organic produce, you are supporting sustainable agriculture. Every time you choose to feed your family and yourself healthy natural

food, you support the return of the food industry back to your grandparents' days of wholesome, hearty, and healthy food.

3. **Support your local farmers' market** or Community Supported Garden (CSG) and local food co-ops. These are grass root folks like you, who are trying to bring healthy food to your table.

4. **Start your own vegetable garden**. Some vegetables grow well even in pots. Fruit trees are easy to grow in some areas of the country. We have a small lemon tree in a pot on our patio.

# What About Organic?

What does the term "organic produce" really mean? The Food and Drug Administration (FDA) standard for organic produce requires that the soil in which organic seeds are planted must be free of herbicides, pesticides and fungicides for one year. Additional standards include no GMO seeds, no sewage sludge for fertilizer, and no food irradiation for preservation. California standards are stricter and require three years of clean soil. There are national and local reputable organizations that offer organic certification to farmers. They have set explicit standards which govern all areas of production. Look for the seal of organic certification on a package or label. Read further for information about labeling for animal proteins such as meat and poultry.

*Organic food industry sales have grown from $1 billion in 1990 to over $55 billion in 2010. Its annual growth is a steady 20% and it represents 4% of all food and beverage sales* *in the U.S. The amount of certified organic agricultural land increased from 914,800 acres in 1995 to 1.5 million in 1997, a jump of more than 60% in just two years.*

## Healthy Soil = Healthy Food

Soil is a living creative mix of minerals, vitamins and decaying organic material. Soil is being recycled by a multitude of living organisms, from microscopic to earthworms to larger burrowing animals. This soil community must be nourished like any living organism.

Organic farmers use soil-enriching natural methods such as crop rotations. They utilize natural compost created from organic matter. They plant nitrogen-fixed cover crops such as clover or soybeans. They also integrate pest management and apply balanced minerals to keep conditions at their best for a natural growth cycle.

Once harvested, organic produce is minimally processed, packaged, stored, and transported to retain maximum nutritional value. This is done without artificial preservatives, waxes, colorings, or other additives, irradiation, or synthetic pesticides. This is sustainable farming for a sustainable world, and yet government farm subsidies actually discourage proven and sustainable farming practices.

Why wouldn't you want the safest and healthiest food for your family? This motivates me, as a mother, to buy organic food whenever and wherever I can. Is it more expensive? Some foods are, but others are comparable. However, when I compare the cost of getting sick, losing time from work or school, and medical bills to the cost of organic food it becomes a bargain.

> *Nothing is more important to me than my health and my family's health. I had no medical bills for my children because I put my money and my time into nourishing them the best way I could and it paid off in prevention of illnesses. Every meal you prepare is an opportunity to improve your family's health and your own.*

No amount of vitamins or mineral supplements can substitute for nature's intricate balance of nutrients. Often overeating and weight problems are caused by a diet lacking in essential nutrients.

> *Americans are one of the most overfed, but undernourished people in the world. Without good health the quality of life is severely diminished.*

## Fruits and Vegetables

Eat fresh (preferably organic) minimally processed fruits and vegetables for a vibrant life. Fresh vegetables and fruit are essential to a healthy diet as they offer us the vitamins, minerals and enzymes not found in cooked protein and fats. Include several servings of fresh fruits and vegetables daily adding them to lunch, dinner and snack preparations. Frozen, canned or commercially available fruit or vegetable juices are not a substitute for freshly prepared produce.

In an ideal world, we would all have the time and land to grow our own food, pick it when it is perfectly sun ripened at its peak and eat it raw or lightly cooked to enjoy the most nutritious and best that nature has to offer. The great majority of us don't live in this ideal setting and have to rely on farmers to bring us their freshest produce. The freshest will always be found at your local farmers' market as it is usually picked the morning of the market or the day before. Beyond purchasing the freshest produce you can buy, you are supporting your local economy and community.

The next freshest would be to shop in local stores that carry produce they purchase from the local farmers. How do you know which ones do? Just ask where it was grown. I live in California and found that a local health food store was buying organic broccoli from Maine because it was cheaper. This happens all the time. So by the time the broccoli gets onto his produce shelf it is already five to seven days old and has traveled over 3,000 miles. In fact, most of our produce has traveled 1,500 miles and is a week old before it gets to the shelf.

Foods that can be preserved with waxes and sprays, or food that can be picked un-ripened and ripened later (like bananas and tomatoes) can be shipped from anywhere in the United States. Food is not grown for taste or nutrition, it's grown to to be shipped thousands of miles and still look "fresh" when it gets to the grocer's shelf.

# Selecting and Storing Fresh Fruits and Vegetables

When choosing fresh fruits and vegetables, the two most important factors are quality and ripeness. If you use all your senses carefully, you will be able to select the produce that is the freshest and ripest.

## First, Look for Characteristic Color, Shape and Appropriate Size.

**Color**—the color should be intensely deep and appropriate to the vegetable. Green zucchini should be very green. If a vegetable looks pale by comparison to others, it was either picked too early (not as much flavor) or allowed to grow too large so it contains more water. Eggplant should be a deep purple/black. Fruits should have rich color to them as well. Basically, if the color attracts you, and it looks delicious to you before you even prepare it, it's probably the right color.

**Size and Shape**—Large size doesn't equate with the best flavor. For instance, because of the seeds, it is best to pick vegetables such as cucumbers, eggplant and zucchini that are thin rather than fat; winter squash on the smaller size rather than the larger. Pick smaller summer melons, as they will be sweeter. Feel for the weight—the heavier, the more juice, the fresher it is. I look for smaller peppers as well as they tend to be more flavorful.

**Feel the Produce**—Is it too hard or too soft? Ask the grower or produce manager how to pick a ripe vegetable or fruit. Cucumbers, eggplant, winter and summer squashes should be firm to the touch and shiny. Ripe tomatoes and avocados should give slightly when touched. Additionally, the fruit or vegetable should have a natural shiny coat to it and not because of wax that has been applied. Fresh foods from farmers' markets are not waxed or treated with sprays, so they may not look as shiny as their supermarket cousins.

**Smell the Produce**—Some fruits such as peaches, melon and pineapple have a mild scent when they're ripening. However, most vegetables will not have a noticeable odor to them even when ripe.

**Storing**—Once you've brought your produce home, you need to protect its freshness and flavor. Most vegetables will need to be kept in a plastic produce bag and then put in the vegetable crisper in your refrigerator. There are green cellulose bags available in most health food stores that do a good job of extending the life of your produce.

Some fruits should be stored at room temperature as the cold temperatures of a refrigerator can damage the flavor. Pears, bananas, citrus, mangos, papayas and pineapples ripen quickest on the counter. The only fruits that I refrigerate if I am not going to eat right away are berries, cherries and grapes. It is best to consume fruit within two to four days and vegetables within four to six days. Longer storage results in the loss of flavor and freshness. So buy local, buy fresh, eat fresh.

Avocados and tomatoes, both fruits, technically, do best on the counter in their own basket. Once avocados are ripe, however, refrigerate them to extend their life. I never refrigerate my tomatoes as they only get sweeter as the days go by. They can last up to a week or longer in the basket on my kitchen counter. Make sure the basket is away from direct sunlight and don't leave produce in plastic bags on the counter. Moisture and carbon dioxide collect and can lead to over-ripening and decay. If you have purchased produce such as bananas and want to hasten ripening, place them in a paper bag with a ripe apple for one to two days.

## Store These Fruits and Vegetables Properly

### Store in the Refrigerator

**Fruits**—apples, apricots, blackberries, figs, blueberries, cherries, grapes, pears, strawberries and raspberries.

**Vegetables**—Artichokes, asparagus, green beans, lima beans, beets, Belgian endive, broccoli, Brussels sprouts, cabbage, carrots, celery, cauliflower, cut vegetables, green onions, herbs (except basil), leafy vegetables, peas, spinach, summer squash, sweet corn

### Ripen on the Counter First—then refrigerate

**Fruits**—avocados, kiwifruit, nectarines, peaches, pears, plums

### Store only at room temperature:

**Fruits**—bananas, grapefruit, lemons, limes, tangerines, mangoes, melons, oranges, papayas, persimmons, pineapple, plantain, watermelon

**Vegetables**—Cucumbers, dry onions, eggplant, garlic, potatoes, pumpkins, winter squash, sweet potatoes, tomatoes, peppers

## Raw vs. Cooked

Your diet should consist of 30-40% raw vegetables and fruits and 25% cooked vegetables. Enzymes are found in raw vegetables and fruits and are essential for optimal good health. However, enzymes are destroyed within minutes of cooking when temperatures are above 114 degrees (almost all cooking techniques). However, cooking more fibrous root vegetables softens the fiber and allows us to absorb more nutrients. So a balance of both cooked and raw is important.

When planning a meal, please include vegetables from each of these categories. They each offer a unique balance of minerals and vitamins necessary for optimum health:

- Under the ground: root vegetables such as carrots, turnips, radish, parsnips, onions, etc.
- On the ground such as broccoli, cabbage, cauliflower, winter squash, etc.
- Above the ground such as leafy greens, peas, peppers, tomatoes, etc.

## Pick the Rainbow

Color is essential in picking nourishing foods too. Fruits and vegetables will have a high amount of particular antioxidants based on their color. So choose some fruits and vegetables from each of these categories:

**Red** fruits and vegetables are colored by a red pigment called lycopene, an antioxidant that has been shown to reduce the risk

of cancer and heart disease and improve memory. Red fruits
and vegetables include cranberries, strawberries, red raspberries,
watermelon, tomatoes, pomegranates, red peppers, beets and red
radishes.

**Orange and yellow** fruits and vegetables
are colored by an orange pigment
called beta carotene. These foods
are abundant in antioxidants,
vitamins, and phytonutrients that
can help reduce your risk of cancer
and delay aging. Orange and yellow
fruits and vegetables include mangos,
oranges, peaches, winter squash, corn,
sweet potatoes and carrots.

**Green** fruits and vegetables get their color from chlorophyll.
Chlorophyll molecules have a similarity to human blood.
Chlorophyll aids in gastrointestinal issues, promotes formation
of red blood cells, detoxifies cancer-causing toxins, treats bad
breath, fights infections, and helps assimilate other minerals.
Green vegetables rich in chlorophyll include spinach, collard
greens, green peas, kale, parsley, Swiss chard, turnip greens,
broccoli, sea vegetables, bell peppers, Brussels sprouts, green
cabbage, celery and green beans.

**Blue and Purple** fruits and vegetables are colored by purple
pigments called anthocyanins, disease-fighting phytonutrients.
Anthocyanins help to protect our brains as we age, and reduce
the risk of diabetes, certain types of cancer, and heart disease.
Purple fruits and vegetables include blood oranges, mangosteen

(www.earthsjuice.com), blueberries, black raspberries, plums, purple grapes, eggplant and radicchio.

**White** fruits and vegetables are colored by white pigments called flavonoids. These powerful phytochemicals can help reduce certain types of cancer, balance our hormones and activate natural immune cells. White fruits and vegetables include pears, bananas, dates, onions, garlic, potatoes and cauliflower.

In Summary:

- ➤ Pick fresh, ripe produce.
- ➤ Eat some raw and some lightly-cooked vegetables and fruit.
- ➤ Choose some roots vegetables and some leafy and round vegetables.
- ➤ Pick fruits and vegetables from a rainbow of colors.
- ➤ Choose a variety of vegetables to eat during the week.

# Free Range and Organic Meats

## Food Labels—Read Between the Lines

Many food labels are either unregulated or misleading. Federal regulations don't allow hormones in poultry or hogs. So, the label stating hormone-free on a package of chicken is a standard industry practice. Growth hormones and antibiotics, however, are permitted in the beef industry. So look for no antibiotics or growth hormones on meat labels.

Terms such as "all natural," or "lower in fat," or "good source of whole grains" aren't regulated and are considered volunteer labeling. Ad writers and marketers make sure the labels and packaging convince you, the consumer, to buy their products.

*Natural* for meats and poultry means no artificial colors or ingredients were added to the raw product before packaging. For instance, a turkey labeled "natural" would not be allowed to have colored fat injected under the skin so it roasts more golden.

*Free Range* applies to poultry and it simply means that the birds were allotted a specific amount of space to "roam" within the confines of their coops. There may be a small fenced-in area for some outdoor "pecking." This limits the number of birds a rancher can put in his hen house. By the way, an average hen house is the size of a football field and can house over 100,000 birds. Access to the outdoors is optional and allowed only during limited times.

One leading U.S. organic poultry brand affords their birds five square feet of outdoor area. The National Organic Standards Board Livestock Committee is proposing that USDA organic standards reduce the outdoor area to just two square feet layer and one square foot per broiler! This is no better than the current industry standard for factory farms, and certainly inadequate for organic farming. Eggs from organic free range hens raised outdoors are far more nutritious than eggs from commercially raised hens.

*Grass-fed* meats are also referred to as free range and require that the animals be allowed to graze outside the confines of the barn.

This definition does not guarantee that the animals were fed organic feed or were spared antibiotics and growth hormones. Generally speaking, most ranchers who label "grass-fed" will also label "hormone-free."

***Organic*** standards for chicken or other meats have stricter guidelines. The animals must be free range or grass-fed, antibiotic-free, growth hormone-free and most importantly, they are fed organically grown feed, hay, etc. These are the "cleanest" choices for healthy protein.

## Fresh Eggs or Aged?

Laying hens usually molt for three to four months out of the year. During that time they normally lay very few eggs. Commercial egg production requires a steady supply of eggs, so chickens are raised in overcrowded conditions and are forced to lay eggs throughout the year, yielding poor quality eggs.

How do you tell if an egg is fresh? Drop it in water and it should sink to the bottom. Why? Because a fresh egg has only a small "air cell" between the albumen and the shell, not enough to let it float. The older an egg, the more it dehydrates and the larger this air pocket becomes. If the egg is submerged, but is suspended, it's not fresh but you can use it safely. If the egg completely floats to the top, throw it out.

A fresh-farm egg will take a little effort to crack as the shell should be thicker than you are accustomed to seeing. It will also have a deep yellow colored egg that stands up high when placed into a pan. There will be a tight bubble of albumen surrounding the yolk and there will be very little water runoff. Go to *www. SuzanneLandry.com* for a video comparison of egg quality.

Oh, and by the way, there is no nutritional difference between brown or white eggs. It simply is the color that a particular breed of chicken lays. Long Island Reds (auburn-feathered chickens), lay brown eggs and White Leghorn hens lay white eggs. It's psychological, I know, but I too prefer brown eggs.

Compared to commercially produced eggs, organic eggs have:

- 4 to 6 times as much vitamin D
- 1/3 less cholesterol
- 1/4 less saturated fat
- 2/3 more vitamin A
- 2 times more omega-3 fatty acids
- 3 times more vitamin E
- 7 times more beta carotene

# Not Milk?

You will find very few recipes in this book that include dairy ingredients for several reasons.

- Food can be delicious without added dairy.
- Most dairy available is pasteurized and devoid of beneficial enzymes.

- Most dairy comes from cows fed rBGH growth hormones.
- Reducing dairy consumption automatically reduces dietary cholesterol and saturated fats.
- Many Americans suffer from health problems due to dairy consumption.

A balanced diet that includes calcium-rich foods should give you enough calcium. I raised my now adult sons without dairy and they are 6'4", 6'3" and 6'1" in height. Clearly, they got enough calcium in the natural food diet on which I raised them. Two-thirds of the world's population doesn't eat dairy food and suffers no ill affects. However, I would recommend you seek the advice of a holistic practitioner or nutritionist before eliminating dairy completely from your family's diet.

If you read my introduction, you know that all my sons suffered from allergic reactions to cow's milk. Identifying food allergies or intolerances and then treating them through dietary changes is not the standard Western medical approach. The medical profession is primarily geared toward treating diseases and symptoms. After all, the American Dairy Association spends hundreds of millions of advertising dollars convincing you and your doctor that milk is the best source of calcium and we need it to stay healthy.

# Dairy Allergies

Lactose intolerance is the most common food allergy. Actually, it is less of an allergy and more of a food intolerance and malabsorption problem. Most of the world's population is not biologically designed to digest milk of an animal other than their own mother's milk. Pasteurization renders it further indigestible.

> *The biological purpose of cow's milk is to provide large amounts of energy and nutrients to grow a calf from 60 pounds to 800-1,200 pounds within two years. To support that growth, cow's milk contains more protein and calcium than human milk. Human milk will contain a higher amount of carbohydrates for proper brain growth.*

What we think of as common health problems are likely due to pasteurized milk intolerance. Most people cannot digest cow's milk because it contains more than 25 different indigestible proteins. These can induce adverse reactions such as eczema, asthma, colds, allergies, ear infections, headaches, lethargy, fatigue, muscle pain, irritability, restlessness, hyperactivity, and mental depression. Worse yet, in some, it can contribute to diabetes, ovarian cancer, prostate cancer, osteoporosis, bone disease, Crohn's disease, constipation, and weight gain.

The late Dr. Benjamin Spock discouraged parents from feeding their children what he referred to as "cow glue."

> *Casein, the protein of milk, is also used as*
> *a raw material in commercial glue, paint,*
> *plastics and dental materials.*

Casein is one of two proteins found in milk and forms a ball in the stomach. It may "gum up" the intestinal walls and may block nutrient absorption in some people. According to a study by the American Academy of Pediatricians, "Since cow's milk protein can irritate the lining of the stomach and intestine, leading to loss of blood into the stools, this can lead to iron deficiency anemia in children. In addition, cow's milk lacks the proper amounts of iron, vitamin C, and other nutrients that infants need. Cow's milk also does not contain the healthiest types of fat for growing babies. Human milk contains a natural balance of vitamins, especially C, E, and the B vitamins, so if you and your nursing baby are both healthy, and you are well nourished, your child may not require any supplements of these vitamins."

## Got Hormones?

Most commercial dairy products come from farms that use a genetically engineered recombinant bovine growth hormone called rBGH. This hormone is produced by genetically engineered bacteria and can increase milk production by three to five times. A cow is injected every 14 days for 200 days of their 335 day lactation cycle, keeping the cow in a perpetual cycle of gestation and lactation, thus extending the length of milking time.

Cows are already overproducing milk. In 1930, the average cow produced 5 kilograms (kg) of milk per day, but by 1988, milk production was at 18 kg a day. With rBGH injections cows can produce and average of 22 kg per day! This is not the way nature intended cows to produce milk.

This kind of milk production wears out the cows' bodies quicker, and an expected life span of 20-25 years is reduced to five years or less. Stress also causes mastitis (udder infection) necessitating the addition of even more antibiotics to their feed. Stress further reduces birth rates so fewer calves are born. It becomes a vicious cycle.

Are there hormones in your milk? You bet! Milk contains not only residues of rBGH as mentioned above, but also excessive amounts of estrogen. Cows treated with growth hormones (rBGH) require more energy-dense food. This is provided by adding meat and bonemeal to their feed, derived from rendered animals from slaughterhouses, increasing risk of *mad cow disease*. Add to this milk shake: antibiotics, rBGH hormone, pesticide residues, pus from the infections and potential bacteria such as salmonella, staphylococci, listeria and deadly E. coli. Now, I ask you, does this sound like a safe and healthy food for you and your family?

The Center for Science in the Public Interest has reported that 38% of milk sampled in 10 U.S. cities is contaminated with antibiotic residues (30 to 60 different types) and sulfa drugs. This increases human tolerance to most antibiotics, which may lead to digestive problems and yeast overgrowth. So, if you choose dairy, even occasionally, buy organic! Organic standards do not allow the use of rBGH, growth hormones or antibiotics on cows.

# Milk Substitutes

I don't recommend most of the many soy products that mimic dairy and meats on the market. To start with, 90% of soybeans are genetically modified. Additionally, soybeans go through some pretty extreme manufacturing to get them to the "just-like-meat" stage. Soybeans weren't eaten as a food crops until 1100 B.C. when fermented soy came into use.

Some of the possible concerns are enzyme inhibitors, phytic acid and hemagglutinin, which are present in soybeans. The best forms of soy to eat are either fermented like miso, tempeh, or soy sauce, or sprouted soybeans. Tofu goes through very little processing and is fine for most people. Please always look for organic soy products to avoid GMO.

There are a variety of cheeses and milks made from rice and almond milk or grain milks that are delicious alternatives. Most of them, however, do not contain sufficient amounts of calcium.

# Non-Dairy Calcium Foods

Many green vegetables have absorption rates of more than 50 percent, compared with about 32 percent for milk. In 1994, the American Journal of Clinical Nutrition reported calcium absorption to be 52.6 percent for broccoli, 63.8 percent for brussel sprouts, 57.8 percent for mustard greens, and 51.6 percent for turnip greens. The calcium absorption rate from kale is approximately 40 to 59 percent. Likewise, beans (e.g. pinto beans, black-eyed peas, and navy beans) and bean products, such as tofu, are rich in calcium if it contains calcium sulphite as an ingredient.

Green leafy vegetables, beans, calcium-fortified non-dairy milks, and calcium-fortified 100-percent juices are good calcium sources with advantages that dairy products lack. They are excellent sources of phytochemicals and antioxidants, while containing little fat, no cholesterol, and no animal products.

| Food Source | Serving | Amount |
| --- | --- | --- |
| Alfalfa | 1 Cup | 10 mg |
| Almond Butter | 2 Tbsp | 86 mg |
| Almonds | 1/4 Cup | 89 mg |
| Azuki Beans, Boiled | 1 Cup | 63 mg |
| Baked Beans | 1 Cup | 128 mg |
| Beet Greens | 1/2 Cup | 82 mg |
| Blackeyed Peas | 1 Cup | 42 mg |
| Bok Choy, Cooked | 1 Cup | 158 mg |
| Broccoli, Boiled | 1 Cup | 94 mg |
| Broccoli, Raw | 1 Cup | 42 mg |
| Brussel Sprouts | 1 Cup | 46 mg |
| Butter Beans | 1 Cup | 40 mg |
| Calcium-Fortified O.J. | 8 Ounces | 300 mg |
| Carrots, Raw | 1 Medium | 19 mg |
| Chick Peas | 1 Cup | 77 mg |
| Chinese Cabbage, Boiled | 1/2 Cup | 79 mg |
| Collards, Boiled | 1 Cup | 357 mg |
| Dried Figs | 10 Figs | 269 mg |

# Salt of the Earth

Table salt is made up of sodium, chloride, and potassium which are minerals our body needs. These are electrolytes that work with carbon dioxide to maintain the acid-base balance in your body, to keep the proper balance of body fluids, and to transmit nerve impulses. So unless instructed by your health care professional, do not eliminate salt completely from your diet. If you eat many meals at fast food restaurants, or consume snacks or junk foods, you are getting more salt than you need for your daily dose. There is more salt on one potato chip than I use in an entire pot of rice for my family! In one can of store-bought soup, there is an entire day's recommended allowance of sodium! So read your labels and limit salty snacks and processed foods.

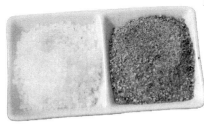

I am frequently asked why I think sea salt is better than kosher or common table salt. Table and kosher salt is at least 97.5% sodium chloride, and there are significant differences in the origin and processing of these salts. Sea salt contains more trace minerals. The textures are different and professional cooks prefer one over the other depending on the dish prepared.

**Sea salt** is harvested from evaporated seawater and it goes through little or no processing, leaving its minerals intact. These minerals flavor and color the salt. Sea salt is not the best salt for canning or pickling as the minerals tend to cloud the water.

Although the government requires that all salt sold for table use contains at least 97.5% sodium chloride, sea salt may contain trace minerals such as: calcium .40%, potassium .12%, sulfur .11%, magnesium .10%, iron .06%, phosphorus .05%, iodine .002%, manganese .0015%, copper .001%, and zinc .0006%. These amounts are very small, but the American diet is overly processed and deficient in trace minerals. I believe that whenever we can, no matter how small the amount, we should eat foods that contain trace minerals, and that would include the use of sea salt.

**Common Table Salt** is mined from underground salt deposits. In processing, a small amount of aluminum hydroxide or calcium silicate is added to prevent caking. This salt is flash-heated to over 1,200 degrees and then crystallized. Table salt is the name for sodium chloride. I don't consider this a healthy salt to consume on a daily basis. The RDA (recommended daily allowance) for sodium is 2,400 milligrams, but most Americans are consuming two to three times that amount.

**Iodized Salt** is table salt that has iodine added. Added iodine is important in areas where a local diet is lacking in iodine-rich foods such as fish and seafood. Dextrose is added to stabilize the iodine and keep the iodine from evaporating. Otherwise, it is similar to common refined table salt.

*The fine grains of a single teaspoon of table salt contains more salt than a tablespoon of kosher or sea salt.*

**Kosher salt** is a coarse flake that takes its name from its use in the koshering process. Kosher salt is particularly useful in preserving and curing meats because its large crystals draw moisture out of foods more effectively than other salts. Some brands of kosher salt contain yellow prussiate of soda, an anti-caking agent, but unlike the anti-caking additive in table salt, it doesn't cloud pickling liquids. It can be derived from either seawater or underground sources. Kosher salt is preferred in restaurants since its coarse texture is easier to use when seasoning dishes. Sea salt's cost prohibits its widespread use in most restaurants.

**Salt Substitute** is often used by people who are on a sodium-restricted diet. It's made from potassium chloride and contains no sodium. It may not be a healthy choice for people who have kidney problems or other ailments where excess potassium can be harmful. Always consult with your health care professional when making major changes in your diet.

**Lite Salt** is a sodium chloride and potassium chloride mixture. Lite salt has 50% less sodium than regular salt and may have iodine added.

# The Real Scoop on Sugar

Who doesn't love sweets? I prefer fruit-based, homemade desserts occasionally over chocolate. Whenever I mention to people that I don't crave chocolate and I could do without it, I get a startled response. We all have our preferences and being aware of the quality of sweeteners can help you choose healthier alternatives to the "addictive white poison—sugar."

## What is Sugar?

Sugar is a simple carbohydrate: a chemical compound composed of carbon, hydrogen and oxygen atoms in a 1:2:1 ratio. Digestive enzymes reduce all carbohydrates to glucose (called blood sugar) for absorption. Whether we are eating brown rice or brown sugar, the end result will be blood glucose. So why eat brown rice when the end result is the same glucose? When we understand how our bodies process carbohydrates, the answer becomes clear.

Whether carbohydrates are simple or complex, their main dietary function is to supply cells with energy. It is the speed at which carbohydrates turn into blood glucose that is important. Carbohydrates that convert quickly are referred to as high glycemic. Refined, simple carbohydrates cause a sudden rise in blood sugar alerting the pancreas to release insulin to transport sugar to the cells. This excess glucose is converted into fat energy for later use. The more refined a sweetener (such as white and brown sugar) the quicker and higher the glycemic effect on the blood and insulin levels. For more information about the glycemic index, refer to the section *Glycemic Index and Carbohydrates* in Chapter 2. You may also do an internet search for "glycemic food chart."

Carbohydrates such as whole grains will digest more slowly causing a gradual rise in blood sugar without a "sugar rush" and the resulting insulin reaction. This gives us needed energy for hours without the "sugar blues" that often follow the use of refined sweeteners.

## How Sweet it Is! Sugar Blues

According to the U.S. Department of Agriculture (USDA), Americans are consuming 156 pounds of sugar and sweeteners per person, each year! Most of this excess sugar is in the form of high-fructose corn syrup (60%). According to the World Health Organization (WHO), consumption of HFCS, which flavors everything from salad dressings to condiments, crackers, snacks and soda has increased 3.5% per year in the last decade. That's twice the rate at which the use of refined sugar has grown.

- Soft drinks contain the greatest amount of HFCS. Our consumption of soft drinks has more than doubled since 1985 — from ten gallons per person a year to more than 25 gallons.
- Most of this HFCS is added to refined, processed and junk food. You wouldn't imagine that yogurt, peanut butter, ketchup and some types of crackers are loaded with hidden sugar, but they are. Always read labels.
- Between 1987 and 1997 sugar consumption increased another 20% during the low-fat and no-fat diet craze. Consumption of added sugar in processed baked goods increased due to manufacturers replacing sugar instead of fat for flavor and Americans gained an average of 8.5 pounds.
- Bone fractures in adolescents have increased by 34%. This is due, in part, to adolescent increased consumption of soda, decrease in milk consumption

and very little water. Soda accounts for twice the volume of milk in an average child's diet. Soda contains phosphoric acid which can interfere with calcium absorption in the bones. Both the soda and lack of water can lead to a chronic acidosis condition which will further leach calcium from the bones and teeth.

The United Nations and the World Health Organization released guidelines in 2003 that say sugar should account for no more than 10% of daily calories. In a 2,000-calorie-a-day diet, that amounts to 200 calories, or only eight heaping teaspoons of table sugar! A single can of regular soda has the equivalent of 10 teaspoons! Check labels, because once you start paying attention, you will be shocked to learn that sugar and HFCS is everywhere! Buyer beware as the manufacturers and marketers of HFCS have now changed the labeling to read simply "corn syrup" (no doubt, a more user-friendly term).

**High Fructose Corn Syrup** is made by an additional refining process using a GMO (genetically modified organism) bacteria for fermentation. It is a very common ingredient in processed foods and beverages and has been recently linked to diabetes and obesity. HFCS will also be labeled as high fructose corn syrup, glucose syrup, corn syrup, and dextrose. HFCS has a glycemic index of 87, while white table sugar is 100! Avoid all high fructose corn syrup products.

**White sugar** is made from either sugar beets (30%) or sugar cane (70%) that has been refined and processed, resulting in 99.9% sucrose. By the way, sugar beets are one of the more recent patented GMO seeds approved for planting by the FDA.

Additionally, white sugar causes a very high glycemic reaction in the blood.

White sugar lacks the vitamins, minerals, fiber, protein and trace elements that were present in the natural plant from which it was processed. *Sugar is loaded with empty calories!* When you eat an excess of sugar, your body must borrow vital nutrients such as calcium, sodium, potassium, and magnesium from healthy cells to metabolize the incomplete food. Over time, calcium loss can result in teeth decay and bone loss eventually leading to osteoporosis. Refined sugars cause a high glycemic reaction in the blood, setting off an insulin response that can lead to weight gain. Read more in the section *Glycemic Index and Carbohydrates* in Chapter 2.

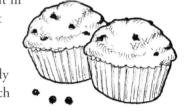

**Brown Sugar** is white sugar with a bit of molasses added back in for color and texture. Brown sugar has no significant nutritional value over white sugar.

**Turbinado** or **Raw Sugar** is made the same way as white sugar except for the last extraction of molasses. It still contains 96% sucrose with very little nutritional value.

**Natural Sweeteners** are your best choice and can actually have some nutritive value, because they are made from natural whole food sources with very little processing. Natural sweeteners are digested more slowly and won't cause the glycemic spike and drop in our blood sugar ("sugar blues") as dramatically as refined sweeteners. Natural sweeteners have varying degrees of sweetness and glycemic reactions, so experiment with them. Most are great for baking, but depending on their liquidity, you might have to adjust your recipe for texture. Diabetics must be very cautious when using any type of sweetener. We are all familiar with honey, maple syrup and molasses, but many others such as agave, date sugar, Rapadura (evaporated cane sugar), rice syrup, barley malt, yacon syrup, sorghum and fruit juices are all unrefined and so retain valuable nutrients. These sweeteners can be purchased in health food stores. Most of these sweeteners have a low glycemic effect on your blood sugar.

Here are a few healthy substitutes:

- **Stevia** is an herb with highly concentrated sweetness and has a "0" glycemic effect.
- **Agave** syrup is made from agave cactus (same cactus used in tequila) and is similar to honey but is milder and half as sweet. Also a low glycemic.
- **Brown Rice Syrup** is malted syrup from brown rice and is less sweet than honey.
- **Barley Malt** is a malted syrup from barley, similar to but milder than molasses.
- **Honey**, especially raw honey (unheated in processing) is an excellent and healthful choice.
- **Pure Maple Syrup**—Born on the east coast, I have to admit this is my favorite.

# Chapter 2

## Getting the Nutrition You Need

Nutrients needed in a healthy diet consist of four groups:
protein, fats, carbohydrates and vitamins/minerals. In addition,
our bodies need trace minerals, enzymes and
clean water. Most foods have a
combination of all of these nutrients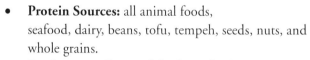
in a greater or lesser degree. It is
necessary to get a variety of these
nutrients from your food selection.

- **Protein Sources:** all animal foods,
  seafood, dairy, beans, tofu, tempeh, seeds, nuts, and
  whole grains.
- **Fat Sources:** all animal foods, seafood, eggs, dairy,
  beans, avocados, seeds, whole grains, nuts, and vegetable
  oils.
- **Carbohydrate Sources:** whole grains, breads, pastas,
  beans, cereals, flours, vegetables, and fruits.
- **Vitamins and Minerals:** all foods in varying degrees,
  but fruits and vegetables are two of the best and highest
  sources of these nutrients.

So let's take these by each category and look at the quality of
nutrients that are best for a healthier diet.

# The Importance of Protein

The word "protein" is derived from the Greek root word
meaning "of first importance." Protein is the basic material of
life. Excluding water, protein constitutes three-quarters of our
body tissues. Organs, muscles, some hormones, enzymes and
antibodies are largely composed of protein.

The basic structure of protein is a chain of amino acids. There
are 22 amino acids identified as the building blocks of protein.
Proteins are constantly being broken down, reused, replaced and
rearranged with infinite possibilities. This process is known as
protein turnover and goes on throughout life. However, there are
only 13 of these amino acids that our bodies make. That leaves
nine of them considered "essential" and necessary to obtain from
our diets.

Foods that contain all the essential amino acids are considered
complete proteins. Complete proteins will always be found
in animal food and their by-products such as dairy or eggs.
Those that don't contain all essential amino acids are considered
incomplete proteins. Incomplete proteins found in grains, beans,
vegetables and fruits need to be combined with other proteins
to help the body utilize all the amino acids. If you are following
a vegan or vegetarian diet, please see my next section *Protein
Combining for Vegetarians.*

➢ Animal food is usually about 15-40% protein by weight. Excessive amounts of animal protein can decrease calcium in the body and put greater stress on the kidneys.

➢ The protein content of cooked grains and beans ranges from 3-10%.

➢ Most vegetable and fruit protein is lower than 3%.

➢ Soybeans and nuts have protein contents comparable to meat, but soybeans themselves are difficult to digest. This is why fermented soybean byproducts such as tempeh, miso and soy sauce are more digestible and healthier.

➢ Although high in fat, nuts are a good source of essential fatty acids and protein. This fat is unsaturated and is considered a good fat.

Peanuts are a legume, not a nut, but highest in protein. Commercial peanut butter contains hydrogenated oils that are added to increase the shelf life. Most commercial peanut butter is 47% fat! Almond butter, lower in fat than peanuts, contains some calcium, has an alkalizing effect on the body and is a delicious alternative.

Government estimates show that the typical American is consuming twice as much protein as the RDA. Our protein needs are easily met with 20-35% of our total caloric intake.

## Protein Combining for Vegetarians

All meats, poultry, seafood, milk, cheese, eggs, quinoa and cooked soybeans are called complete proteins because they contain sufficient amounts of all nine essential amino acids that we must obtain from our food.

Whole grains, beans, legumes, nuts, seeds, vegetables and fruit are foods that contain incomplete proteins. If you are a vegan or a vegetarian, you should have a wide variety of all these foods throughout the day. Combine the following in your day's meal planning or within a day's meal and you will increase your overall protein and nutrients:

**Whole grains with any bean**—Try chili over brown rice or with cornbread or tofu over brown rice, quinoa or a whole grain tortilla with beans. See my *Black Bean and Garden Vegetable Enchiladas* or *Hot Tamale Pie with Red Beans* in the *Bean Cuisine* chapter of *The Passionate Vegetable* (go to *www. ThePassionateVegetable.com).*

**Beans with any seed or nut**—For example, try *Hummus (Chickpea) Spread* containing sesame tahini, which can be served with whole grain crackers or in a pita sandwich.

**Whole grains with dairy**—Try grated cheese over steamed vegetables and *Chicken Parmesan* in *To Meat or Not to Meat* or *English Rice Pudding* in *Good for You Desserts* all in *The Passionate Vegetable.*

**Whole grains with any seed or nut**—Try *Rocky Road Rice* or *Bulgur Pilaf with*

*Mushrooms* in *Amber Waves of Grain* chapter found in *The Passionate Vegetable.*

**Beans with dairy**—Add grated cheese over chili in my *Vegetarian Chili* in *Bean Cuisine* chapter found in *The Passionate Vegetable.*

# Pick Your Protein

| Food | Amount | Calories | Protein | Carbs | Fats | Saturated Fat | Cholesterol |
|------|--------|----------|---------|-------|------|---------------|-------------|
| Beef/Pork | 8 oz | 614 | 40 | 0 | 48 | 20 | 156 |
| Chicken | 4 oz. | 260 | 32.8 | | 13.2 | 3.7 | 48 |
| Bass | 4 oz. | 141 | 26 | 0 | | 2.9 | |
| Cod | 6.8 oz | 377 | 25.9 | 0 | 29.5 | 95 | |
| Shrimp | 4 oz | 112 | 23.7 | 0 | .3 | 221 | 10 |
| Cream Cheese | 1 oz | 60 | 3 | 2 | 5 | 3 | 10 |
| Yogurt | 8 oz | 100 | 13 | 13 | 0 | | |
| Almonds | 1 cup | 836 | 28 | 29 | 74 | | |
| Sunflower Seeds | 1 cup | 821 | 32.8 | 27 | 71 | | |
| Pinto Beans | 1 cup | 230 | 17 | 42 | 1 | | |
| Red Beans | ½ cup | 120 | 7.3 | 22 | 2.0 | | |
| Garbanzo Beans | ½ cup | 134 | 7.3 | 22 | 2.1 | | |
| Tofu | 1 oz | 22 | 2.3 | .5 | 1 | | |
| Avocado | 1 oz | 46 | .6 | 2.1 | 5 | 78 | |
| Soy milk | 8.4 oz | 140 | 10 | 14 | 4.6 | | |
| Rice | 1 cup | 232 | 4 | .49 | 1.2 | | |
| Oatmeal | 1 cup | 87 | 7.9 | 25 | 2.3 | | |
| Egg | 1 poached | 74 | 6.2 | .6 | 6.5 | 212 | |

Since many vegetables contain small amounts of protein, you can see it is quite easy to get protein in a vegetarian meal. It has been my experience that most vegetarians don't get enough protein and other vital nutrients to stay healthy because they haven't been as careful to combine protein foods in a wide enough variety. Many eventually return to a meat-based diet because they don't feel as healthy as they expected. There are other factors, of course, including digestion and absorption problems that can lead to low protein in vegetarians. Hopefully, you have found a health care practitioner that can guide you through a transitional diet. Take cooking classes too!

# Clarifying the Fat

Understanding healthy fats vs. unhealthy fats can be less confusing if you remember that there are three major forms of dietary fat:

> - *Unsaturated Fats* are liquid at room temperature and are considered healthy fats. Unsaturated fats are mostly made up of polyunsaturated or monounsaturated fats. High quality organic expeller pressed oils are your best choice and are found in health food stores. These oils are found in quality vegetable foods such as nuts, seeds, grains and beans.
>   - *Monounsaturated fats include olive oil, peanut oil, almonds, avocados, sunflower oil, sunflower oil (high oleic) and canola (rapeseed) oil and lard.*

- ○ *Polyunsaturated fats include soybean, corn, walnut, hemp, grape seed, safflower, sunflower (linoleic) and flax oils.*

➢ *Saturated Fats* are solid at room temperature and should be eaten in moderation. They are found in animal proteins, tallow, suet, all dairy foods, butter and tropical fats, such as palm kernel oil and coconut oil (more to follow on coconut oil and butter). Saturated fats are stable and do not become rancid when subjected to high heat.

➢ *Trans Fats and Hydrogenated Fats* are the result of high heat specialized processing and are considered one of the unhealthiest fats. They rob oil of nutrition leaving it virtually indigestible and carcinogenic, and they potentially raise blood cholesterol. Virtually all commercial oils, except olive oil, are processed this way. I strongly recommend you replace these oils with expeller pressed oils found in health food stores (refer to the section *Trans Fats: The True Villain*).

So, the healthiest and the most delicious oil to use in food preparation is extra virgin olive oil (more on that later) and a light expeller pressed oil such as sesame oil.

## Unsaturated Fats

Unsaturated fats are by far your best choice for oils in your diet. Vegetables oils make up the majority of oil that is unsaturated.

To further understand unsaturated fats, I've listed the best of them.

- ➤ **EVOO—Extra Virgin Olive Oil** is the best of the best and the most nutritious grade of all olive oils. Light olive oils are refined and less nutritious. They are made from the same virgin green olives used for the extra virgin oil, but they are mixed with a chemical solvent to pull more oil out of the same olives. Then they are pressed again. This process is repeated three times! The combination of all these pressings results in light olive oil. Light olive oil is an inferior product in taste and nutritional value. When I want a lighter oil flavor in my dishes I use one of the other oils mentioned above.

- ➤ **Flaxseeds, Chia Seeds and Hemp Seeds** all are great sources of Omega-3. They are high in protein, soluble fiber, and alpha-linolenic acid (ALA). ALA is an Omega-3 fat that is a precursor to EFA, which is the fat found in fish oil. Flaxseeds are concentrated sources of lignans and phyto-nutrients that modulate hormone metabolism. They also have potential anti-cancer properties, especially for colon and breast cancers.

Flaxseed oil should not be heated. Instead use it in salad dressings or drizzle on vegetables or in oatmeal. It is best to grind flaxseeds at home yourself (using a designated coffee grinder) and store in the refrigerator for a few days. Always store flaxseeds and flaxseed oil in the refrigerator.

- ➤ **Omega-3 EFA** (essential fatty acids) are essential to be obtained from our food. Research shows that Omega-3 is an anti-inflammatory that promotes blood flow. Additionally, it lowers the risk of heart disease, arthritis, and cancer. Many modern diseases begin with chronic inflammation. The best food sources for Omega-3 include salmon, sardine, herring, swordfish, green mussels, halibut, anchovy, mackerel, tuna, organ meats, egg yolks, flaxseed oil and flaxseeds, chia seeds and hemp seeds.

➤ **Omega-6 EFA** (essential fatty acids) promote blood clotting and reduce inflammation. Today, eggs and animal food contain more Omega-6 than Omega-3. When animals were grass fed, their meat contained a higher amount of Omega-3. It's interesting to note that the Alaskan Inuit people have a 1:1 ratio of Omega-3 to Omega-6. This is because they eat equal portions of seafood and land animals such as caribou. They also have extremely low incidences of most modern diseases. In comparison, most Americans are getting a 1:15 ratio of Omega-3 to Omega-6. No wonder we have so many inflammatory-based diseases!

## Saturated Fats

➤ **Butter vs. Margarine**
One tablespoon of butter contains 11 grams of total fat. A whopping 7 grams is saturated with 30 mg of cholesterol and is 10% of your recommended daily fat allowance! Butter has shortcomings but contains no trans fats. If it's made from organic milk, it is even less processed. Pasteurization kills all of the beneficial

enzymes found in raw milk. Read more in my section *Not Milk* in Chapter 1.

Margarine was formulated in 1869 as a viable low-cost substitute for butter. Dubbed oleomargarine, it started with softened beef fat to which salty water, milk, and margaric acid was added. By the turn of the century, the beef fat in the original recipe was replaced by vegetable oils. It was sold as a white spread and it wasn't until 1950 that the production of yellow margarine began.

Margarine is processed in a similar way to chemically extracted hydrogenated oils. To make margarine into a spreadable product, pulverized nickel is used as a catalyst to turn a liquid fat into a solid fat. As of this writing, most margarines still contain trans fats and have been hydrogenated. Read your labels! Almond or other nut butters are a better choice for your morning toast.

➢ *Tropical oils* are emerging as desirable, less-expensive alternatives to hydrogenated fats. In the late 1980s, tropical oils (coconut, palm, and palm kernel) were shunned because they are high in saturated fat. Now nutrition experts find that they may not be as bad as once thought.

➢ *Coconut Oil,* although a saturated fat, more than half of it is lauric acid which has many health benefits. It also doesn't have the same effect on cholesterol as other fats. Coconut oil is considered antimicrobial, antioxidant, antifungal and antibacterial. It has a high smoking point so many people enjoy using it as their primary cooking oil. Personally, I don't like all my food tasting like coconut, but some love it!

➢ ***Palm Oil*** or palm fruit oil comes from the pulp of the palm fruit. It contains a significant amount of heart-healthy monounsaturated fats, vitamin E, and antioxidant compounds. Research now indicates that palm oil behaves like an unsaturated fat in the body— that is, it may help reduce blood cholesterol levels.

➢ ***Palm Kernel Oil*** is more saturated than palm oil and contains little monounsaturated fat. Less is known about palm kernel oil; it is often further processed (fractionated) to reduce the liquid portion. This leaves behind more saturated solids. You may have noticed "fractionated palm kernel oil" as an ingredient in several energy bars and other reformulated products. This makes the coatings less likely to melt. It isn't known if this processed oil is any better for you than hydrogenated fats.

***This doesn't mean these oils get a green light. How they're processed is still questionable and their quality is still debatable.***

# Chemical Extraction vs. Expeller Pressed Oils

The way oil is extracted greatly affects its nutritional quality. Oils are either chemically extracted or expeller pressed. Chemically extracted oils are most commonly referred to as hydrogenated oils. These oils are the majority of the commercial oils typically found in your local grocery store.

## Chemical Extraction

To extract oil from seeds, grains, or nuts (all having a hard coating) the commercial oil extractor first soaks these seeds in hexane, a petroleum solvent. The solution is then boiled at high temperatures to evaporate the hexane and release the oil. This damages the quality and taste of oil.

> *At high temperatures the oil converts from essential fatty acids into trans-fatty acids. Trans-fats have been shown to raise cholesterol levels and increase free radicals in the blood. Not healthy! Additionally, the high heat begins to spoil the oil giving it a shorter shelf life due to rancidity.*

Under federal regulations, food-grade oils must be shelf stable for one and a half years. To prevent rancidity and to accomplish this, these oils are hydrogenated, a process by which the oil is passed through hydrogen gas, resulting in sticky, thick and gray oil. The soluble materials are then removed with different processes including degumming (removing phosphatides), alkali refining (washing with alkaline solution to remove free fatty acids, colorants, insoluble matter, and gums) and bleaching (with activated carbon to remove color and other impurities.) Frankly, it sounds like it might be better oil for my car than my body!

None of this is clearly labeled, but is simply stated as "pure vegetable oil." How misleading! My teenage sons would break out in pimples within days after indulging in friends' junk food and snacks. This oil is simply not digestible.

**Expeller Pressed Oils** (which I recommend) are mechanically pressed after soaking the product in a saline solution. They are superior in taste and quality. This method brings a smaller yield at a higher cost. However, it is a small price to pay for greater health. Since these oils are not hydrogenated, they have a shorter shelf life, usually three to six months. It is best to keep them refrigerated to retain freshness. You can leave a small oil bottle near your stove and refill as needed. Oils give rich flavor and moisture to dishes and shouldn't be eliminated. Vegetable oils provide the essential fatty acids that many Americans lack in their diet.

Heating any oil to high temperatures for deep frying will damage the quality and health benefits. Deep frying anything doesn't fall into the category of healthful eating, but if you do occasionally, use a light expeller pressed oil labeled for high heat cooking.

## Trans Fats: The True Villain

For years the dietary fat villain had always been saturated fats. New evidence points to trans-fatty acids (trans fats) as the real villain.

Harvard University researchers reported that in a study of people who ate hydrogenated oils (high in trans fats) had nearly twice the heart attacks as those who did not. They reported that replacing trans fats with unsaturated vegetable oils could prevent at least 30,000 heart disease deaths in the U.S. each year.

Small amounts of trans fats are found naturally in meat and dairy foods. But trans fats found in processed foods contain partially hydrogenated oils. Processed foods include many baked goods, snack foods, margarines, microwave popcorns, frozen meals, even some peanut butters and most snack foods.

Hydrogenated trans fats are created by chemical extraction process. This process is referred to as RBD, (Refined, Bleached and Deodorized) and contains unnatural polymers and carcinogens unfit for human consumption. It makes food crispy, creamy, moist, and flavorful and shelf stable—the most important consideration in our profit-conscious food industry.

Fast food is often fried in partially hydrogenated oil because the oil stands up well with repeated use. But the trans fats that result behave like saturated fats in your body. Trans fats raise both total cholesterol and LDL (bad) levels. Additionally, trans fats lower protective HDL (good) cholesterol. They may also increase triglycerides and inflammation and have been linked to an increased risk of diabetes.

Saturated fats and trans fats have been linked to elevated levels of cholesterol, so exercise caution with these foods. The standard recommendation is to reduce saturated fats by reducing portion sizes of meats and dairy or by choosing low-fat dairy.

> *All fats regardless of processing have about the same amount of calories, so use all fats in moderation, especially if you're concerned about weight gain.*

# Navigating the Carbohydrate Maze

Refined carbohydrate consumption has skyrocketed and saturated fat consumption has decreased, but Americans are still battling the bulge. Overconsumption of refined carbohydrates is a contributing factor to our growing obesity problem. If you are confused as to which carbohydrates are good for you (complex carbohydrates) and which are not (refined carbohydrates), it's time to clear the confusion.

All carbohydrates (both refined and complex) are energy foods because they metabolize into blood sugar called glucose. Glucose circulates in our blood and provides energy to all our cells. Carbohydrates differ in their nutritional value and in how quickly they convert into glucose. This conversion of carbohydrate to blood glucose is measured by the glycemic index. More on that later in this section.

At rest, our brain requires two-thirds of our body's total glucose needs! The brain cannot store fuel so it requires a constant supply of glucose. When glucose blood levels fall too low in the brain, some people may experience temporary mental fatigue or dizziness. During exercise, our muscles use glucose for quick energy. Once limited glucose reserves are gone, the body will break down muscle to provide our brain and muscles with glucose.

To meet our energy needs while preventing muscle loss, complex carbohydrates can be included in our diets to provide needed glucose.

## The Glycemic Index and Carbohydrates

Before we can understand the value of complex carbohydrates over refined carbohydrates, we need to understand the glycemic index. Basically, the quicker a carbohydrate is converted into usable blood glucose, the higher its glycemic index. The slower a carbohydrate is digested and converted into blood glucose, the lower the glycemic index, which is more desirable.

A sudden rise in blood glucose (high glycemic reaction) from eating candy, for example, causes the pancreas to release insulin. Insulin is a storage hormone directly responsible for removing excess glucose from the bloodstream and storing it as glycogen and then later as fat. So eating high glycemic foods, refined carbohydrates (see below), too often will lead to fat storage in the body. Additionally, when insulin levels in our blood rise, they block the release of fat-burning glucagon. Simply put, eating an excess of carbohydrates, even fat-free carbohydrates, will prevent your body from burning stored fat. This is not a formula for weight loss!

## Refined Carbohydrates

Refined processed carbohydrates, the "bad" carbs, contribute to weight gain, obesity, insulin resistance, metabolic syndrome, type two diabetes, food addictions, overeating, and many diet related diseases.

Refined carbohydrate sources include the more commonly eaten white flour products, including breads, pastas, cereals, crackers, cookies, desserts, sodas, sugars, candies, pastries, donuts, bagels etc. Read more in the section, *The Real Scoop on Sugar*, in Chapter 1.

Refined processed carbohydrates are the worst part of the Standard American Diet (S.A.D.). These foods might be all right to eat occasionally, but are downright addictive if eaten frequently. These are all high glycemic carbs and will cause an undesirable blood sugar spike. Combining the occasional refined carbohydrate side dish with foods containing fiber, fat or protein can help to lessen its blood sugar rush.

## Complex Carbohydrates

Complex carbohydrates, the "good" carbs, will digest more slowly because they still contain fiber and protein. Complex carbohydrates include whole grains, beans, vegetables, fruits, some dairy and natural sweeteners.

Fiber and protein both slow down the digestion of all carbohydrates, lessening the glycemic rush of blood sugar. Complex carbohydrates are unrefined and still retain their fiber (bran) and protein. On the other hand, there is usually little to no fiber and very little protein in refined carbohydrates resulting in a high glycemic blood sugar.

Can you improve the glycemic of a carbohydrate? Yes, if you combine foods that have protein, fat and fiber in them. So, for example, having a serving of white pasta with marinara sauce would be a high glycemic meal. Instead, choose whole grain pasta with at least 6 grams of fiber and 7 grams of protein per serving. For added protein and fat, serve with a meat sauce, or for vegetarians, add chopped nuts to your sauce. White rice will cause a sudden blood sugar rise because it has been stripped of its fiber, fat and protein (germ and bran). Brown rice, a whole grain, contains carbohydrate starch, protein, fat and fiber, all of which helps to slow down a blood sugar rise. Having brown rice with beans or nuts adds more fiber, fat and protein, further slowing down the glycemic of these carbohydrates.

Eliminating all carbohydrates from our diet is radical and unhealthy, but you can make smarter choices. I suggest you limit your consumption of refined carbohydrates and experiment with complex ones. Make whole grains an essential part of your healthy meal planning. You will find more than fifty recipes for whole grain cooking, plus a cooking chart, in my *Amber Waves of Grain* and *Salads that Satisfy* chapters in my cookbook, *The Passionate Vegetable.*

# Healthiest Water for Cooking and Drinking

Your **most essential** nutrient is water. You are 70% water, so why not drink the best? No discussion of healthy living can be complete without a discussion of the quality of water you drink. The type and quality of water for drinking, to wash and to cook your food is important because the contaminants and properties of water are absorbed into your foods. Tap water, depending on where we live, may contain chlorine, minerals, and undesirable contaminants such as rust, sediment, organochlorides like trihalomethanes, lead, hydrogen sulfide, barium, cadmium, arsenic, fluoride, nitrates, benzene, etc. Washing organic produce in chlorinated water simply contaminates your produce. That's not an ingredient in any of my recipes!

*"Cancer risk among people drinking chlorinated water is as much as 93% higher than among those whose water does not contain chlorine."*

U.S. Council of Environmental Quality

*"Each day, millions of Americans turn on their taps and get water that exceeds the legal limits for dangerous contaminants."*

USA Today-Special Report,
"How Safe Is Your Water?"

Good water can help you achieve excellent health and vitality. If you are fortunate to have your own deep well water and live in a pristine, clean environment, you may want to skip this chapter. Apparently most of us don't, because bottled water sales have soared over the past few years. A more economical approach to better drinking and cooking water is to purchase a filter and do it yourself. Most good filters will remove some to all of the contaminants listed above. Please consider improving your water quality to be a top priority for a healthy lifestyle.

> *We are made up of 70% percent water! Our cells are bathed in, surrounded by it and made up of water. Doesn't it make sense to use the cleanest water possible?*

## Water pH—Is It Important?

Our blood must maintain a pH balance between 7.35 to 7.45 always. Anything below 7 is acidic and above 7 is considered alkaline. If we, however, eat an acidic diet the pH of the fluid in our tissues becomes more acidic. Chronically, this can lead to diseases and mineral loss. So, it's important to eat a more alkaline diet (75% plant food and 25% animal) and drink water that is alkaline.

The alkalinity of water will depend on the amount of alkaline minerals vs. acidifying minerals. For instance, calcium is alkaline and chlorine is acidifying yet both are found in ordinary water. The pH of tap water is neutral, roughly around 7 pH only because lye is added to municipal water to balance the corrosive chemicals (such as chlorine) to prevent rusty pipes (not your body pipes—their pipes).

In nature, water from streams and rivers (presumably unpolluted) will vary from 6.5 to 9.5 in pH. So, when deciding on water the pH is as important as the "cleanliness" of the water. Most bottled water is pretty acidic and sodas . . . OMG . . . extremely acidic.

## Bottled Water—What You Don't Know

In March of 1999, the Natural Resources Defense Council (NRDC) released a report called "Bottled Water, Pure Drink or Pure Hype?" This report points out that 60% to 70% of all bottled water is completely exempt from the FDA's bottled water standards, because it is bottled and sold within the same state. Unless the water is transported across state lines, there are no federal regulations that govern its quality!

> *The Natural Resources Defense Council report concluded that, "Therefore, while much tap water is indeed risky, having compared available data, we conclude that there is no assurance that bottled water is any safer than tap water."*

By the way, I have tested the pH of every bottled water we could find and the majority of them are acidic from 4.5 to 6.5 pH with a few that are a neutral 7.0 pH. Before I truly learned about the quality of water, I was drinking reverse osmosis water to which I added some trace minerals. I thought I was bringing up the pH by increasing the minerals, but when we tested the water it was still very acidic at 5.5 pH!

The reality of bottled water is that you pay from $1 to $4 a gallon for the perception of higher quality, when in fact the quality of bottled water is at best unknown. Quality home water treatment is by far the most economical in the long run, the most convenient, and the best way to enjoy truly healthy, great-tasting water. It is also the right choice environmentally!

What about our landfills? It's estimated that 80% of the 28 billion petroleum-based plastic water bottles purchased every year land up in our landfills. Not to mention that bottled water manufacturing created more than 2.5 million tons of carbon dioxide. Oh, and biodegradable? Yes, but in about 1,000 years!

Bisphenol A (BPA) and phthalates found in these plastics find their way into the water we drink, especially when left in a hot car or in storage crates for too long. The plastics used in these disposable bottles are endocrine disruptors. Some of this water was bottled over a year ago! These toxins have been found to cause fatigue, weight gain and hormone imbalances.

## Are You Drinking Away Minerals?

Tap water can be purified by carbon filters, reverse osmosis, and distillation. However, the best water filtration method is electrolyzed (ionized) water. While filtration methods mentioned below may remove undesirable taste and most of the contaminants such as chlorine, detergents, parasites, pesticides, bacteria, viruses and cancer-causing chemicals, some can also remove beneficial minerals such as magnesium, calcium, potassium, etc.

Water produced by these filtration methods is called "dead" water because the water produced tends to be acidic, has large water clusters and free radicals (oxidizing) known to accelerate aging and cause disease. Drinking this water can cause the body to deplete minerals found in our bones, teeth, muscles and other internal sources to maintain an alkaline blood. This is counter-productive for optimal health, well-being, adequate hydration, and slower aging. Below are examples of some of the more common filters that are available.

## Choosing a Filter

- **Granular Activated Carbon Filters** create an increased surface area that can absorb many of the toxic chemicals and organisms found in tap water. Activated carbon filters can trap bacteria without destroying it. So solid carbon filters are preferred.
- **Reverse Osmosis** (R.O.) will remove most of the remaining contaminants as stated by the manufacturer's specifications but, also removes essential minerals. R.O. uses pressure to push water through a membrane filter to remove contaminants. The resulting R.O. "dead" water is also acidic.
- **Distillation** removes contaminants by boiling water to produce a vapor which is collected and cooled back into 99.9% pure liquid water. This "dead" water is also devoid of essential minerals and is acidic.

## The Best Water

- **Electrolyzed (Ionized) Water** is produced by a water ionizing machine. After water is filtered, it goes through the ionizer device. Unlike the above filters, the machine separates the water into acidic water and alkaline waters. The alkaline water contains minerals and is micro-clustered (groups of five to six water molecules per cluster) which brings out the flavor in the foods, cooks food faster and has a negative charge which means it has antioxidant properties. To read how important acid/alkaline pH is in our diet, see *Acid-Alkaline Balance*. Your water quality is just as important.

This sounded like the best choice for my family, so I researched different ionizers. I found and purchased a medical grade water ionizer device from Japan manufactured by a company called Enagic, Inc. The company was started in 1975 and is the only original equipment manufacturer (OEM) with an impressive list of industry certifications and awards unmatched by any other water ionizer company. The water produced by their machine is so unique that Enagic was granted a trademark by the U.S. government for *Kangen Water™*.

I bought their top selling model, the SD501, with a full 5 year warranty, and I expect it to last me 15-20 years. To learn more about Enagic machines and quality comparisons, visit www.LivingWaterforLife.com or follow the link on www. suzannelandry.com. If you want to research, start by researching the international manufacturer's credentials and Gold Standards of Enagic, just as you would in choosing a board certified doctor.

Choose quality over price when it comes to your health and getting results.

## Improved Health

Do I feel an improvement with this water? Oh, yes! Always trying to drink more water to keep myself hydrated, it seemed I was also spending an equal amount of time in the ladies room, feeling that I wasn't absorbing it. Now, I feel hydrated and my skin and hands are soft and my nails are getting harder! I'm a chef with perpetually soft nails and dry skin. My husband's sinuses are clearing after years of childhood congestion and we are both sleeping better. Weight loss is happening for two friends of mine as they drink more alkalized water. I know personally three people had their eczema disappear after topically using this water for a few weeks.

## How much water should we drink?

I recommend that you drink half your weight in water per day. So, if you weigh 150 pounds drink at least 75 ounces or roughly two-and-a-half quarts of water. It is easier to drink this volume of ionized water because it tastes delicious. You can count fresh vegetable juices and herb teas in this volume of water but not caffeinated beverages, which are very acidic and dehydrating. For optimum health, drink 8.5 pH water, which is an option on these ionizers.

# Chapter 3

## You Are What You Digest

Of course, the popular saying "everything in moderation" certainly has some validity. There are many factors besides stress, life changes and emotional upsets that rob our energy and vitality. Excessive heavy protein and fats, caffeine, sugars and sodas, processed foods, hydrogenated fats and excessive fried foods will absolutely slow you down. Unless you're 18 years old, the days of eating a hamburger and fries at 1:00 A.M. and still feeling good in the morning is long gone!

Allergies, poor digestion, malabsorption, and improper food combinations rob energy too. If you feel dragged out and exhausted in the morning without your cup of java, then something is lacking in your overall diet or lifestyle. If you had a good night's sleep you should feel energized in the morning without the caffeine.

For most of my first 28 years I had been a "slow starter" in the morning. I shuffled instead of walked and grunted instead of talked, and it was only after one or two cups of coffee, around 11:00 A.M. that I came alive. My mother is the same way, so we accepted it as a family characteristic and I adjusted my lifestyle, becoming a night owl. Never did I expect that changing my diet would affect these morning doldrums, but almost instantly I felt better in the morning. Previously there were mornings when I woke up more tired than I had been when I went to bed. Sound familiar to you? I simultaneously eliminated red meat, coffee and sugar from my diet and started to eat whole grains. For the first time in my adult life, I felt energetic, awake, and alive in the mornings. With a diet that was well balanced and nourishing, I found that I could better handle the life challenges presented to me.

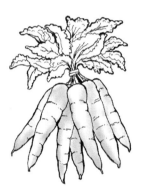

You will learn in time what foods your body best functions on, digests easiest, provides you with the most energy, and gives you satisfaction and nourishment.

Digestion is affected by more than our food combining so please keep in mind these important points:

- Avoid eating a heavy meal when you are emotionally upset, stressed or right after exercise.
- Eat only when you are hungry. Stop before you are full. It takes 20 minutes for satiation (sense of fullness) to take effect. Eat slowly so that you feel satisfied on less.
- Don't eat late dinners. Digestion needs three hours to empty your stomach. A full stomach will compromise a good night of sleep.

- If you must eat a late dinner, choose vegetables served with pasta or a whole grain for dinner. Eat your heaviest proteins and fats at lunch.
- Drink little or no liquid (especially cold water) with meals. Liquids dilute digestive juices and slow digestion. Wait 45 minutes after a meal to resume drinking fluids.
- Eat slowly, putting your fork down between each bite. Relax and breathe as you chew.
- Chew each bite of food at least twenty times before swallowing. Chewing is a process, not a race.
- Follow good food combining practices (read further).
- Stay hydrated during the day by drinking ½ oz. of water per lb. of body weight.
- Include foods such as yogurt, kefir or pickled vegetables such as sauerkraut, cucumber pickles, etc. to help increase intestinal "flora."
- If you are over 40 years old or have trouble digesting foods, include a good digestive enzyme with every meal.

*Keep a positive attitude towards life, yourself and others. Along with a healthy diet, this is the best prescription for a happy long life.*

## Free Radicals and Other Energy Robbers

Free radicals are basically incomplete and highly reactive molecules that attach themselves to cells and the genetic material inside them causing deterioration (called oxidation) leading to cell mutation or cell death. In turn, radicals released from these cells can start a damaging chain reaction to other tissues in the body. Free radicals are believed to play a role in heart disease, cancer, pre-mature aging and overall loss of health and vitality.

Free radicals are produced through the normal process of metabolism. Fortunately, the body is designed to handle a certain amount of oxidation and free radical activity. Today, we are exposed to a much larger amount of damaging free radicals from our environment, indoor and outdoor air pollution, radiation, home cleaning products, personal care products, and cigarette smoke. These place extra toxic loads on our bodies.

The current "standard American diet" consisting of fast foods, unhealthy fats, fried foods, processed food, refined carbohydrates, sugars and excessive meat all contribute to free radical damage. The greatest control we have over limiting free radical damage is through the food choices we make. The antioxidants in foods, especially fruits and vegetables offer us some protection against free radical damage.

# Protective Antioxidant Rich Foods

Antioxidants provide our body protection against free radical oxidation by counteracting or neutralizing free radicals and their destructive effects. Whole, fresh foods are abundant in antioxidant rich vitamins and minerals. There are hundreds of different substances that can act as antioxidants. The most familiar ones are <u>vitamin C</u>, <u>vitamin A and E</u>, <u>beta-carotene</u>, and other related carotenoids, along with the minerals selenium and manganese. They're joined by glutathione, coenzyme Q10, lipoic acid, flavonoids, lycopene, phenols, polyphenols, phytoestrogens and many more.

Vitamins C and E are found in plentiful supply in fresh fruits and vegetables. However, at least 60% of vitamin C is destroyed after ten minutes of cooking. Whole grains, beans, nuts, some meats, poultry and fish also contain some antioxidants.

Although antioxidant supplements are widely available, it is most beneficial to obtain antioxidants through fresh food because your body can assimilate and use the antioxidants from fresh food much more efficiently. Organically grown foods have higher levels of vitamins, minerals and antioxidants than conventionally grown foods.

Here is a list of the top 20 sources of antioxidants in commonly consumed foods per the *"American Chemical Society. Largest USDA Study Of Food Antioxidants Reveals Best Sources."*

Starting with the richest source of antioxidants they are:

- ➢ Small red beans
- ➢ Wild Blueberries
- ➢ Red kidney beans
- ➢ Pinto beans
- ➢ Blueberries (cultivated)
- ➢ Cranberries
- ➢ Artichokes (cooked)
- ➢ Prunes
- ➢ Raspberries

➢ Strawberries
➢ Red delicious apples
➢ Granny Smith Apples
➢ Pecans
➢ Sweet Cherries
➢ Black Plums
➢ Russet Potatoes (cooked)
➢ Black beans (dried)
➢ Plums
➢ Gala Apples

# Super-Foods for Super Health

Some foods are called super foods because they are some of the most nutrient dense foods available and contain other phytochemicals that are found to be protective against disease. There are entire books devoted to super-foods. In fact, just about every brightly colored fruit and vegetable fits the category of a super-food, as do nuts, beans, seeds and aromatic and brightly colored herbs and spices. You can incorporate some in your meal planning while others could be taken as nutritional supplements. Here are some of the best:

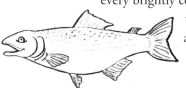

➢ **Wild Caught Salmon**—high in Omega 3
➢ **Green Super-Foods** have the highest concentration of digestible nutrients, vitamins and minerals. These include dark leafy greens like kale, collard greens,

broccoli, spinach and super-greens such as wheatgrass and barley grass for example.

➤ **Beans**—chili beans are one of the best as well as lentils.

➤ **Whole Grains**—quinoa which is highest in protein and gluten free. Barley and oats are among the others.

➤ **Green and White Teas** are both high in antioxidants.

➤ **Fruits**—kiwi (highest in Vitamin C) berries (high in antioxidants), pomegranate and avocados. Super-fruits like mangosteen juice (www.earthsjuice.com) goji, acai and cacao are the highest in antioxidants.

➤ **Nuts and Seeds**– almonds and walnuts are some of the best. Super-seeds include flaxseed, hemp and chia seeds.

➤ **Bee Food** (pollen, honey, jelly) The western world actually discovered the benefits of bee super-foods by accident during an investigation of native Russian beekeepers who regularly lived past 100 years of age and who ate raw honey, rich in bee pollen, every day.

➤ **Seaweeds** (sea vegetables)—hiziki, wakame, kombu (kelp), arame, nori, etc. are the most nutritionally dense plants on the planet containing up to 10 times more calcium than milk and eight times as much as beef. The chemical composition of seaweeds is so close to human blood plasma, that perhaps their greatest benefit is regulating and purifying our blood system.

➤ **Herbs and Spices**— turmeric, curcumin, rosemary,

cinnamon, capsicum found in peppers, aloe vera, ginseng, echinacea and nettle to name just a few. Herbs have been used for centuries as part of the wisdoms of natural healing methods. Herbs as medicine are essentially body balancers that work so the body can heal and regulate itself.

➢ **Fermented Foods** –yogurt, kefir, raw sauerkraut, pickles, sourdough breads, unpasteurized vinegars or acidophilus supplements for extra probiotic support.

# The Vital Role of Enzymes in Digestion

Proper digestion of your food along with the quality of the food you consume is essential. You may eat the highest quality of food available, but if your digestion is weak, the assimilation of those nutrients will be incomplete and you will not derive the healthy energizing benefits of good food.

> *As we age, our digestion functions decrease. So eat more fresh fruits and raw or lightly cooked vegetables in your diet for their enzymes and be more aware of proper food combining. Consistent nourishment offers us consistent energy!*

Before foods can be absorbed through the small intestines and transported to our cells via our bloodstream, they are broken down into simpler biochemical forms. The catalysts that break down the particles of our food into absorbable molecules are called enzymes. Without enzymes we would not be able to make use of the essential nutrients that we eat! Enzymes are vital to our life and without them our bodies would cease to function. Enzymes can be divided into three major categories:

- **Food or Plant Enzymes** are present in all raw plants and are responsible for three functions: pre-digestion, nutritional support, and acute repair. Plant enzymes that are needed to digest food include protease (digests protein), amylase (digests carbohydrates), lipase (digests fat), disaccharidases (digest sugar), and cellulase (digests fiber).
- **Pancreatic Enzymes** are essentially digestive enzymes secreted by the pancreas, but are also found in our mouth, small intestine, and stomach. These enzymes play a vital role in the digestion of our food.
- **Metabolic Enzymes** are made by our body, and are responsible for running our body chemistry. These enzymes are involved in all body processes: breathing, thinking, talking, moving and immunity. There are hundreds of thousands at work in our bodies at all times.

Early humans primarily consumed raw foods rich in plant enzymes. Our digestive systems are not designed to digest the assortment of processed foods that many people eat indiscriminately. Processed foods lack vital nutrients and enzymes which are found in fresh and raw vegetables and fruits. Less than 10% of adult Americans are getting their recommended "Five-A-Day" for fruits and vegetables. Worse yet, less than 5% of children are getting the recommended amount!

Of the few vegetables Americans do eat, they are often processed or overcooked, destroying vital nutrients (like French fries vs. a baked potato).

> **Enzymes are destroyed by cooking temperatures above 118° F, pasteurization, canning and microwaving.**

So you can see why it's essential to add raw vegetables and fruit to your daily diet. Eating a diet rich in raw foods and taking plant enzyme supplements will help replace those needed enzymes. Supplemental enzymes can be used to optimize digestion, absorption and assimilation of food, which can reverse nutritional deficiencies, act as an anti-inflammatory and help detoxify. Speak to your natural health care provider if you are concerned about digestion as there maybe many factors, other than enzymes, affecting your digestion. When any enzyme deficiency is left untreated, food cannot properly be digested and will inevitably result in many health problems. The most common disorders are food intolerances and allergies.

# Food Combining for Optimal Digestion

There are three macro-nutrients that need to be broken down into absorbable nutrients in the digestive system: proteins, fats and carbohydrates. Each is digested by separate enzymes or acids and will take different times to digest along different areas of the digestive system.

Starches begin their digestion in our mouth and complete the metabolic breakdown in our small intestine. Therefore, starches pass quickly through our stomach for that purpose.

Animal protein begins digesting in our stomach via hydrochloric acid and pepsin. It can take up to three hours for protein to break down in the stomach before continuing to the small intestine where the nutrients are absorbed. Fats digest later when bile is released by the gall bladder.

Because starches pass quickly through your stomach, proteins digest best without starches present. Eating starches with proteins encourages proteins to leave the stomach before they are completely broken down. Proteins may then *putrefy* in the small intestine! This can cause toxic by-products, gas and sometimes indigestion. A build-up of these by-products can result in anything from food allergies and tiredness, to assorted health problems. Don't combine proteins (which require an acid medium to digest) with carbohydrates, starches, sweets or fruits (which require an alkaline medium to digest). So avoid eating fruit for instance with a protein meal. Enjoy fruit (sweet carbohydrate) as an *in-between-meal* snack when you crave sweets or want a boost of energy.

The best carbohydrates to eat with animal protein are vegetables. A meal comprised of a small portion of chicken or other animal protein, cooked vegetables and a small salad will digest easily and your body will feel better for it. If desserts are offered, it is best to wait an hour or more after a meal before eating them. Also, wait approximately 45 minutes to drink fruit juice or water after a protein meal.

Whole grains are a valuable part of a healthy diet. Whole grains, whole grain breads and whole grain pastas are best eaten with vegetables or legumes. Heavy proteins, such as meat, should not be served with whole grains. The principles of food combining are biochemical facts of life and, if respected, will result in better digestion and a healthier you.

> *Although the efforts of changing your dietary habits can present a challenge, the rewards of health and vitality are definitely worth it.*

*In Summary:*

- *Avoid combining protein with carbohydrates, starches or sweets.*
- *Eat your dessert at least an hour after a heavy protein meal.*
- *Don't drink or eat fruit juice or water with a protein meal. Instead, have fruit as a snack between meals.*

# Food Cravings–Getting Off the Roller Coaster

Why do we crave certain foods? Whenever we experience a craving, our body is trying to maintain or restore balance. **When we eat excess salt or protein, we will desire sweets, sodas, alcohol.** For instance, the desire to have a dessert after a meal of animal protein or to have a soda with salty popcorn is a natural response to an imbalance of pH. Our willpower has little to say when our body seeks to balance its blood pH and maintain homeostasis (state of whole-body balance). Please refer to the section *Acidity and Alkalinity* for more information.

Some foods create more "heat" while others are "cooling." The more protein and fat a food contains, the longer it takes to digest. The more energy that is used to digest it, the more heat it produces. Energy creates heat, so, high protein and high fat foods create warmth in the body. That explains why we desire more meats, fats and fried foods in winter seasons or in colder climates.

Vegetables usually digest within one to two hours and fresh fruit within an hour. They produce very little heat during the digestion process. In addition, their higher vitamin, water and sugar content have a cooling effect on our bodies. This explains why we desire more fruits, vegetables, ice cream, sweets, sugar, sodas, hot spices and alcohol in summer and in warmer climates. When our diets are imbalanced with excess proteins and fats and not enough fruits and vegetables, we will crave these cooling foods.

Vegetables, especially dark leafy greens, are high in minerals. *Yet when we are too acidic, the mineral we crave is salt.* It's interesting how eggs taste so much better with a little salt. A centered diet includes foods that are in a balanced ratio of proteins, carbohydrates, fats, vitamins and minerals. An imbalanced meal leads to undesirable snacking which leads to further imbalances.

Plant foods include vegetables, fruits, whole grains, beans, nuts and seeds. It's easier to maintain a healthful balanced lifestyle when each meal is balanced. Keep a 3:1 ratio of plant foods to animal foods on your plate to prevent unwanted cravings.

Food processing destroys nutrients making them empty-calorie foods which throws off our nutritional balance. Antibiotics in meat, artificial preservatives, herbicides, pesticides and growth hormones further take the balance out of food. Is it any wonder that most people don't know what a balanced diet is? Many of my students comment on how well-nourished they feel after tasting the food in my cooking classes. Our shared meals consist of whole grains, beans, fresh vegetables, fruit-based desserts and sometimes sea vegetables. It's almost like our bodies want to say "YES" to healthy food!

> *To get off the food roller coaster, keep your meal balanced with a 3:1 ratio of plant food to animal foods.*
>
> *Consistent good nourishment ensures us of consistent energy and health.*

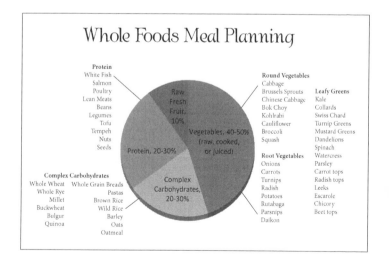

## Whole Foods Meal Planning

**Protein**
White Fish
Salmon
Poultry
Lean Meats
Beans
Legumes
Tofu
Tempeh
Nuts
Seeds

**Complex Carbohydrates**
Whole Wheat    Whole Grain Breads
Whole Rye              Pastas
Millet            Brown Rice
Buckwheat          Wild Rice
Bulgur              Barley
Quinoa              Oats
                    Oatmeal

**Round Vegetables**
Cabbage
Brussels Sprouts
Chinese Cabbage
Bok Choy
Kohlrabi
Cauliflower
Broccoli
Squash

**Leafy Greens**
Kale
Collards
Swiss Chard
Turnip Greens
Mustard Greens
Dandelions
Spinach
Watercress
Parsley
Carrot tops
Radish tops
Leeks
Escarole
Chicory
Beet tops

**Root Vegetables**
Onions
Carrots
Turnips
Radish
Potatoes
Rutabaga
Parsnips
Daikon

Raw Fresh Fruit, 10%

Vegetables, 40-50% (raw, cooked, or juiced)

Protein, 20-30%

Complex Carbohydrates, 20-30%

# Food pH: Acidity and Alkalinity

A healthy body has many buffers that maintain the balance between the alkalinity and acidity of its fluids and tissues. Only a pH balanced internal environment allows normal body function and a strong immune system. Due to our modern lifestyle and the overconsumption of acid-forming foods, we deplete our alkaline reserves. Tissue acid waste then increases, disturbs the pH balance, and leaves our body more vulnerable to disease. Additionally, most Americans do not drink enough water which can lead to acidosis. Refer to *The Healthiest Water for Cooking and Drinking.*

**Acidosis (overly acid diet) can cause such problems as:**

➢ Cardiovascular damage, including the constriction of blood vessels causing oxygen reduction.
➢ Weight gain, obesity, and diabetes.
➢ Slow digestion and sluggish elimination.
➢ Bladder and kidney conditions, including kidney stones. Yeast/fungal overgrowth.
➢ Acceleration of free radical damage, possibly contributing to cancerous mutations and immune deficiency.
➢ Premature aging, low energy, or chronic fatigue.
➢ Osteoporosis, weak, brittle bones, increasing the possibilities of hip fractures.
➢ Joint pain, aching muscles due to lactic acid buildup.

# What is pH ?

The pH is the potential of hydrogen. It is a measure of the
acidity or alkalinity of a solution. It is measured on a scale of
0 to 14. When a solution is neither acid nor alkaline it has a
neutral pH of 7. Less than 7.0 pH is considered more acidic and
above 7.0 pH is more alkaline. The body continually balances its
fluid and tissue pH, with exceptions such as stomach acid, which
is measured at pH <2 for the proper breakdown of protein.

The body continually balances the blood pH to stay between
7.35 and 7.45. If the deviation is pronounced or prolonged
outside these normal limits, *acidosis* or *alkalosis* can occur
leading to disease. Most people who suffer from unbalanced pH
are acidic. This condition forces the body to borrow minerals
(such as calcium, sodium, potassium and magnesium) from
vital organs and bones to buffer (neutralize) the acid and safely
remove it from the body. If this borrowing is prolonged, the
body can suffer severe damage due to high acidity. Deficiency
syndromes, such as osteoporosis, are caused by the body's
ongoing attempts at buffering. Our American diet is too heavy
in acidifying foods: meats, poultry, fish, hard cheeses, coffee,
alcohol, sodas, hydrogenated oils, desserts, sugars, and refined
flour products.

Your body is able to assimilate minerals and nutrients properly
only when its pH is balanced. Without a balanced pH, it is
possible for you to be taking healthy nutrients and yet be unable
to absorb them. If you are not getting the results you expected
from your nutritional, dietary or herbal program, please consult
with a health care professional.

## Bone Loss and pH

A seven-year study conducted on 9,000 women at the University of California, San Francisco, showed that those with chronic acidosis were at greater risk for bone loss than those with normal pH levels. The authors believe that many hip fractures, common among middle-aged and older women are due to a high acid diet, rich in animal foods but low in vegetables *(American Journal of Clinical Nutrition*, 2001*)*.

There is a 34% bone fracture increase in adolescents today due to the overconsumption of sodas in their diet. Many kids today are drinking twice as much soda as milk and hardly any water. The phosphoric acid in the sodas prevents calcium from being absorbed into the bones and less milk means less calcium to counteract the pH imbalance.

## Keeping the Right Balance

Surprisingly, a food's acid or alkaline-forming tendency in the body is not directly related to the actual pH of the food itself. For example, lemons are very acidic, yet the end product they produce after digestion is alkaline. So lemons are actually alkaline-forming in the body. Likewise, meat will test alkaline before digestion, but after digestion meat leaves a very acidic residue in the body. The most influential factors affecting your acid-alkaline pH balance are:

- Dietary choices
- Stress—emotional and physical
- Quality and amount of sleep

- Level of physical activity
- Changes in body temperature

The following is a brief and general list of alkalizing and acidifying foods that will help you with your meal planning.

## Basic Acid-Forming Foods

It is impossible to eat a varied diet that doesn't include at least a few acid forming foods. If you eliminated all acid forming foods, you'd be eliminating all proteins! Acid-forming foods can be 25%-30% of your diet, depending upon lifestyle. These are general guidelines for relatively healthy individuals. If you are in recovery from an illness or surgery, follow the recommendations of your health care practitioner.

| | |
|---|---|
| **Meats** | — all meat, fish, poultry, and shellfish. |
| **Grains and Breads** | — rice, barley, wheat, oats, rye,and corn. |
| **Nuts** | — cashews, walnuts, peanuts, pecans, macadamias and filberts. |
| **Dairy and Oils** | — homogenized milk products, cream, cheese, egg whites, nuts and corn oil. |
| **Legumes and Vegetables** | — lentils, navy beans, kidney beans, adzuki beans and cooked spinach. |
| **Fruits** | — cranberries, blackberries, pomegranates, plums, prunes and rhubarb. |

**Beverages**            — coffee (very acidifying), black tea,
                           soft drinks and alcoholic beverages.
**Chocolate**            — in all varieties.
**Soy products**         — tofu, soy sauce, and miso.
**Sweeteners**           — white sugar and sugar substitutes,
                           brown sugar, milk sugar, cane
                           syrup, malt syrup, molasses and
                           processed honey.
**Oils**                 — flaxseed oil, olive oil, canola oil,
                           evening primrose oil, and borage
                           oil.
**Nuts and Seeds**       — almonds, chestnuts, flaxseeds,
                           sesame seeds, fennel and caraway
                           seeds.

## Basic Alkalizing Foods

Alkaline-forming foods should make up 70-75% of your diet.
Most of these should be vegetables and fruits. Eat at least 50%
uncooked as in salads and snacks. The following is a basic list of
such foods.

**Fruits**    — including citrus,
                apples, pears,
                peaches, blueberries,
                watermelon,
                papaya, mango and
                cantaloupe.
**Vegetables** — sea vegetables
                (seaweed), mustard greens, asparagus,
                parsley, raw spinach, carrots, cabbage, broccoli,

|            |   | potatoes, sweet potatoes, lettuce, onions, garlic and most other vegetables and especially dark, leafy greens. |
| **Grains** | — | millet, amaranth, wild rice, quinoa, buckwheat and sprouted grains (except wheat). |
| **Fish** | — | cold water fish, usually white meat fish. |
| **Dairy** | — | unpasteurized nonfat milk, goat's milk, cottage cheese, plain yogurt, butter and egg yolks. Although I do not recommend dairy foods, they are generally neutralizing. |
| **Beverages** | — | clean or purified water, lemon water, green tea, ginger tea and herb teas. |
| **Legumes** | — | peas, green beans, lima beans and sprouted beans. |
| **Sweeteners** | — | raw honey, raw sugar, maple syrup, rice syrup and stevia. |

In meal planning, it is important to remember to balance alkaline-forming foods with acid forming foods in a 3:1 ratio. If you fill your plate half-full with vegetables (some cooked, most raw) one quarter animal protein and one quarter complex carbohydrates you will maintain that 3:1 ratio. If you add fresh pressed vegetable juice, you'll balance your pH even better.

> *Eat a more balanced ratio of three portions alkaline foods to one portion acid foods. You will become better nourished and feel more satisfied. An added bonus is that you won't experience food cravings and the need for excessive sweets.*

If you desire weight loss, increase vegetables and eliminate whole grains for a while. But if you are craving starches include vegetable starches such as potatoes, turnip, winter squash, carrots, beets and peas along with other vegetables.

Whether you eat alone or with your family, attractive food presentation is important. Make sure your dishes have contrasting colors to create an eye appeal that can't be resisted. A little chopped parsley on top does a lot for a simple bowl of soup. Balance your vegetable, protein and carbohydrate dishes so they offer a variety of textures to your plate. You wouldn't want all your dishes to be soft like mashed potatoes or all chewy either.

I recommend you keep a food journal to record your food choices each day. Recording quantity is less important unless you tend to overeat. You can also record your energy level and mental clarity for that day. I suggest you continue this for at least a month while you are transitioning your diet. After a month go back and read it to see if a pattern emerges between your food choices and how you feel. I guarantee that you will learn something from this exercise that no doctor could possibly tell you!

# Chapter 4

## Begin by Starting

The secret is out—cooking is **not** a mystery. The way to be
a good cook is, well . . . to cook. Just plunge in! The results
don't have to be just right—some of my best dishes were the
result of mistakes or substitutions I made in a recipe.
Even wholehearted efforts sometimes fall short
and the best intentions don't always ensure
success. There is no great secret, only the
experience of doing it over and over again.
Our cooking doesn't have to prove how
talented we are or measure up to some imagined
result. It's your unique way of nourishing yourself
with food.

*Our original worth is not something
which can be measured, increased
or decreased by what we do . . .
especially in the kitchen.*

The more love you put into your cooking, the better your food
will taste. Cooking for yourself or your family is an act of love
because through food you create life. You give your life energy

through cooking to create life again. What a beautiful circle of love! Love is the most powerful ingredient of all. I hope through my recipes, I can encourage you to fall in love with creative cooking.

> *Approach cooking with abandonment and enjoy every morsel of the experience . . . just feed, satisfy and nourish.*

# Food Budgets

Long ago I got the important message from my dad that good health was my wealth. The value of protecting my health was deeply instilled when he died at 47 years of age from a long battle with cancer. So, I put my family's health first, which meant I valued the quality of food we consumed. As a single mom, the routine was to pay rent, make the car and insurance payments and buy food. Everything else could be budgeted.

If I'm in the mood for asparagus or my son asks for red raspberries and the price is high, I buy them anyway. That *desire* is our bodies talking, needing certain nutrients, and when it talks healthy, I listen. Red raspberries are a good source of iron and so my youngest son's love of raspberries was his body telling him he needed iron. I place my priorities on prevention of disease so we are never ill and don't have the need for doctor visits!

*One of the ways I demonstrate love for myself
and my children is through preparing and
eating delicious healthy food . . . despite the
cost.*

I have worked closely with cancer patients for several years now.
I have been blessed to have learned so much from them. One
message that is driven home for me every time is that *prevention
is so much cheaper than the high cost of recovering their health
again.* We've been taught to ignore our bodies' desires. We eat
when we're not hungry, drink water to kill hunger, starve to lose
weight, or follow someone else's schedule for meals. If we honor
our body's language, feed and nourish it, it tells us what we need
and in turn rewards us with health and vitality.

# Making the Transition to Natural Foods

Let's face it, we humans make transitions in our lives very slowly
and sometimes kicking and screaming along the way. So don't
expect your transition to good eating habits to happen overnight.
You've had your present eating habits for awhile, so give yourself
time to change those habits. After all, you may be changing the
tide of ancestral eating habits, not to mention cooking with
ingredients you may have never heard of before.

## Step 1: Begin to Read Labels

The ingredients you use are crucial, so choose the best! My rule of
thumb was simple in the beginning of my transition: if I couldn't
read it, I probably didn't want to eat it. Packaged Danish pastries
(Entenmanns Pecan Coffee Cake *was* my favorite occasional treat

back then) are loaded with unpronounceable ingredients that do not enhance flavor, but just increase shelf life. Buy it freshly baked or bake it yourself and you'll know what goes into it. Ingredients are listed in order of volume first, so if sugar is the second ingredient, watch out! Most commercial cereals average 32-73% sugar!

## Step 2: Substitute Familiar Ingredients

Start eliminating highly-processed food from your diet and substitute natural alternatives. This change alone will affect the overall taste of your favorite recipes and will increase their nutritional value. For example, your favorite dessert recipe can be improved a little by substituting bleached white flour for organic unbleached or whole wheat flour. This way, you are improving the quality of the food you eat without eliminating all the family favorite dishes. For more substitution suggestions, please see *Food Substitution Chart* at the end of this chapter. If your budget is limited, make this transition slowly as you replace pantry items.

## Step 3: Stocking the Pantry

Fill your pantry with basic staples and always have lots of fresh vegetables and fruits on hand to make cooking easier and to be ready when the creative inspiration hits you! Except for buying fresh vegetables and fruits, we could probably live off of what's in our pantry for a month or more. I like it that way. Every grain and bean variety I cook with is in my pantry, along with a wide selection of herbs and spices, pastas, nuts and some prepared

condiments and canned foods. See *Pantry Essentials* in Chapter 5
for a list of suggestions.

## Step 4: Introduce Vegetarian Entrees

Throughout the week introduce a
vegetarian entree instead of a meat or a
dairy dish. Start by introducing a whole
grain side dish a few times a week. If
you are a vegetarian, whole grains are an
important *daily* dish to include in your
meal planning. You can start by preparing
hot breakfast porridge such as cream of rice,
cream of wheat, or oatmeal. Perhaps you'd like
a cold, whole grain cereal instead. I will show you how leftover
grains can be turned into an international selection of new tastes
in my *Amber Waves of Grain* and *Salads that Satisfy* chapters
in *The Passionate Vegetable*. Whole grains are filling and very
nutritious and will help you get off the carbohydrate-craving
rollercoaster.

> *Many of my students have, over the years,
> experienced a drastic drop in their cholesterol
> when they introduced whole grains in their
> diets.*

For the first six months of our transition, I browsed vegetarian
cookbooks for recipes that I made for my family. If we all
enjoyed it and it wasn't time consuming, I would prepare it
again in two weeks. As my repertoire of recipes grew I eliminated
more meat-centered meals. Before very long we were enjoying

our new way of eating. Also, look for ways to present the meat entrees with more vegetables. Instead of steak or barbecued chicken, try beef stir fries or chicken stew with vegetables. This way the portion of animal fat and protein is balanced with more vegetables and your food dollar will stretch serving more people. By the way, you probably won't miss the meat.

## Step 5: Plan Ahead

Eating healthy can take a little more time in preparation, but planning ahead is the best advice I can give. Think of some possible meal ideas for the week and make a shopping list. Having everything on hand makes a huge difference in time preparation for a meal. Having a wide assortment of ingredients doesn't necessarily mean you decide what you'll eat for dinner next Wednesday, but it does give you a general idea of what you can cook during the week.

## Step 6: Saving Time in the Kitchen

This can mean soaking beans overnight (or a few days before) and cooking them in the morning while you are getting ready for work. Cooked beans keep for about five days. You can add some vegetables, herbs or spices to them and in 15 minutes your beans are ready for dinner. Cooked grains will hold for three days refrigerated and so cook them anytime you're at home for an hour or more. For example, tomorrow's grain is cooking on the stove while we are eating tonight's dinner.

If I am planning on making a chicken dish for tomorrow, I prepare the marinade tonight while I am making dinner. I will clean, chop, and bag enough kale or other greens for three dinner servings. While chopping carrots for tonight's stir-fry, I might chop extra for lunches or tomorrow's soup. Sometimes we cook a few more chicken breasts than we need for dinner and turn that leftover chicken into fajitas, tacos, or a Cobb salad for a few quick workday meals.

Try not to let a burner in your kitchen sit idle while you are at home. If you are good at juggling (if you have kids, you definitely are) then you can be cooking on the stove, roasting in the oven, stirring the soup, and chopping all at the same time. Okay, that's a bit much except for a passionate chef like me, but you can eventually learn to coordinate three to four dishes at once.

> *The point is, plan ahead, and when you are in the kitchen keep those hands moving and all those burners going! Just make sure you have all the ingredients on hand and begin prepping!*

## Step 7: Be Playful and Creative

As I said before, some of my best dishes are those that I had no idea what I was going to make when I started looking in the refrigerator and pantry. Once I see what's on hand, the creative juices of possibilities began to bubble in my mind. Experiment! You can always go out to dinner if it is a total disaster. Chances are you will discover a wonderful new dish that may become your new favorite. If you're like me, however, you will be enjoying the creative play so much that you forget to write down the quantities of the ingredients you used. Some of my best dishes never quite got duplicated because of that.

# What Your Taste Buds Know

Our taste buds recognize five basic flavors: sweet, salty, sour, pungent and bitter. More than 80% of our tastes buds are dedicated to sweet flavors. We are hard wired for this propensity because baby's first and most essential food is sweet mother's milk. Beyond the experience of enjoying the taste of food, our brain is stimulated to command the digestive system to get to work.

Chinese medicine understands that certain flavors stimulate respective internal organs. So if you eat something sweet, the organ responsible (pancreas) for maintaining blood sugar levels is activated in response to the intake of this potential sugar.

- Sweet would be any sweet vegetable such as carrots, onions, squash, parsnips or natural sweetener. These are said to stimulate stomach and spleen.
- Salty would be meats or vegetables like celery or condiments such as soy sauce or miso. Believed to stimulate the kidneys and bladder.

- Pungent (or hot) would be onions, ginger, garlic, radish, mustard, horseradish or scallions. Believed to stimulate the lungs and large intestines.
- Sour would be vinegar, lemon, limes, Swiss chard, sour grapes or apples. Purported to stimulate the liver and gall bladder.
- Bitter would be bitter greens like broccoli rabbe (also called rapini), dandelion, kale, mustard greens and turnip greens. Said to stimulate the heart and small intestine. Bitter is one of the most important flavors to have although needed in very small quantity for it is said to stimulate the small intestine and improve digestion.

Isn't it interesting that the two biggest addictions people have are for bitter foods? No . . . not greens! Coffee and chocolate are bitter without the sugar and cream. It's no wonder people love a cup of coffee after a meal (bitter stimulates the small intestine where most nutrient absorption takes place).

> *A meal is more exciting and satisfying if it includes at least three of the five flavors— salty, pungent, sour, sweet and bitter. These flavor dynamics help make a meal memorable.*

In meal planning, try to include a variety of flavors. A little sour can be added to the meal in a salad dressing. Sweet is the easiest to get naturally; just be sure to use a few sweet vegetables or a bean. Salty is also very easy to taste in most meals. Celery is naturally salty tasting. If you eat sea vegetables they are also naturally salty. Pungent can be added with the addition of raw scallions to garnish a soup or grain. If you ever had a meal and still felt *unsatisfied*, it may have been because it lacked flavor dynamics.

# Cooking with Herbs and Spices

The transition to healthy eating can be a delicious experience if you learn to season with herbs and spices. Adding a few, helps dishes pop with flavor while cutting down the need for salt. Even a simple dish becomes special and elegant with the addition of some favorite herbs and spices. The fine art of seasoning can be easy when you use a few guidelines. As with many art forms, appreciate the process and you are more likely to appreciate the results.

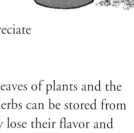

**Herbs:** These are the flower buds and leaves of plants and the flavors are more delicate than spices. Herbs can be stored from six months to one year after which they lose their flavor and color. Basics to keep on hand: basil, oregano, thyme, parsley, rosemary, dill or mint if you wish.

**Spices:** These are from the parts of the plant richest in flavor: stems, nuts, barks, seeds and roots. Spices can be stored for up to three years before losing their flavor. Some spices are hot while others are sweet. Cinnamon, nutmeg or cumin are considered sweet spices and cayenne, chili and ginger are hot. Basic keep-on-hand spices are: ginger, cinnamon, cayenne *or* chili *or* hot red pepper flakes, cumin, and black pepper. If you are wondering why I didn't mention garlic it is because it is technically not a spice or an herb but a bulb, which like onions, shallots and chives, is a member of the lily family.

**Substitution:** When substituting fresh herbs for dried you should increase the quantity by three. When substituting dried for fresh in a recipe, you should reduce by a third. You can be more generous with milder herbs such as basil because I don't think you can ever have too much basil, or garlic for that matter!

**Storage**: Store dried herbs and spices at room temperature away from heat, light and moisture. Fresh herbs, such as parsley, cilantro and dill can last over a week when stored in the refrigerator. Place in a wide-mouth glass jar, fill with water and place a loose bag over top. Change the water every two days and they will remain fresh.

## Cooking Tips:

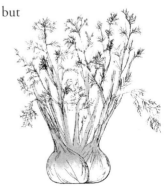

- ➤ Salt sometimes enhances flavor, but excessive salt can easily drown out delicate flavors and leach out important nutrients from vegetables.
- ➤ Add whole spices (such as a cinnamon stick) at the start of cooking to allow their flavor to permeate the food.

➤ Add ground spices midway through cooking; always start off with small amounts when using hot spices and build up to taste.

➤ When blending herbs with dressings or sauces that will not be cooked, blend an hour before needed to let flavors meld.

➤ To increase the flavor of dried herbs, crumble them between your fingers to release their oils and aroma before adding them to your dish.

➤ To use fresh herbs, when the recipe calls for dried, you can use one tablespoon of chopped fresh herbs for every teaspoon of dried herbs.

## Flavor Families

Some herbs and spices complement each other well. They form "flavor families" and can be used together to enhance flavor. Here are some winning flavor combinations:

**Sweet**—allspice, anise, cinnamon, cardamom, cumin, cloves, nutmeg. Use in breads and desserts, especially fruit based pies and fruit breads.

**Hot**—chili peppers, cayenne, garlic, radish, onion. Although fresh cilantro is not hot, it has a unique flavor and is used to cool down hot spices. These flavors are a must in Mexican, Cajun and Spanish dishes. Use in seafood, poultry, soups, salads, marinades and in bean dishes.

**Spicy**—cinnamon, ginger, pepper, star anise. These have a zing to them and are wonderful in Chinese stir fry, soups, poultry, meats, seafood dishes and whole grain dishes such as *Chinese Fried Rice* in *Amber Waves of Grain* chapter in *The Passionate Vegetable*.

***Pungent***—celery seed, cilantro, cumin, curry, ginger, black pepper. Curry blended here in America is less spicy. You can adjust the "heat" to your taste by increasing the amount of cayenne or ginger. Use these spices in poultry, shellfish, meats, beans, whole grains and vegetable dishes.

***Herbal***—basil, parsley, dill, marjoram, rosemary, thyme and sage. These herbs are the basis for a great sauce. Use these herbs for flavoring sauces, gravies, poultry, soups, herb breads, stuffing and muffins.

***Hot spices have a cooling affect on the body. That's why they are popular in countries with hotter climates.***

## Survival Dining for Vegetarians

Eating out can be challenging when you are transitioning your diet. But there are enjoyable dishes you can find to fit into your diet at the home of a friend, on airplanes, or in restaurants.

Visiting with families who eat differently from you does not have to be a stressful experience. If it is for one meal, ask them to prepare a pasta entrée (or bring it yourself). If their entree doesn't fit into your diet, you can always eat the vegetable side dishes that are usually offered with an entree. The biggest challenge for some people is telling family members that they don't want to eat what has been served. You may feel you might hurt their feelings. An easy alternative, if you need one, is to explain that you have allergies or you are doing a food elimination diet recommended by your doctor. If your visit is for several days, I recommend bringing some vegetarian protein sources to heat up without a lot of fuss. For example, frozen veggie burgers or canned beans travel easily and you can purchase tofu almost anywhere. Once your protein needs are taken care of, you can share and enjoy the vegetable and starch side dishes your family will be serving.

Another situation where you may feel your diet is challenged is during air travel. The few remaining airlines that offer meals at all usually have a vegetarian offering. It seems that airline caterers haven't caught up to the idea that whole grains and beans or tofu should be part of a vegetarian meal. If it is a long flight, I will carry on several snacks including nut mixes and fruit to tide me over.

An everyday challenge for some is eating in restaurants. If you're a vegetarian it is even more of a challenge. However, many ethnic restaurants serve vegetarian dishes that include acceptable protein entrees. Eating foods of a different culture can be both enjoyable and festive. My favorite is Japanese restaurants where I get the sea vegetables, vegetables and rice that I love (many of them serve brown rice). Chinese restaurants offer tofu entrees and Mexican restaurants have bean entrees or soups. You'll also find vegetarian entrees in Indian restaurants.

You can get a vegetable salad, cooked vegetables or pasta any place in the world, but after a meal or two, you may need some protein to meet your nutritional needs. Carrying some mixed nuts along with you is a good way to add protein to your diet if beans, tofu or fish are not available. If you eat out frequently, choose a restaurant that offers healthier choices of protein with lower fat content. When eating a fish entree at a restaurant, avoid deep fried entrees. Additionally, order a large salad and for a starch, order a side of rice or a baked potato instead of bread. Yes, and either skip the dessert or share with a friend. My husband and I will occasionally share a fruit-based dessert when we eat out.

## Adapting Your Favorite Recipes

One of the easiest steps to transitioning your diet is to upgrade the quality of ingredients in your favorite recipes. In this way you are taking a step in a healthier direction without causing a mutiny at home. See my *Food Substitution Chart* below for exchanges.

# Food Substitution Chart

| Reduce or Omit | Substitute | Other Changes |
|---|---|---|
| Bleached cake flour | whole wheat pastry flour or organic unbleached white | requires a little more liquid |
| All purpose flour | whole wheat flour or other whole grain flours | requires a little more liquid |
| Processed cereals | whole grain cereals, granola, hot whole grain cereals | |
| Crackers or rice cakes | whole grain crackers | |
| White rice | brown or wild rice, or other whole grain | |
| Cornstarch | arrowroot powder, organic cornstarch or kuzu | |
| Baking powder and soda | low-sodium, aluminum—free baking powder | |
| Common table salt | sea salt, kelp, or soy sauce | season to taste— may require less |
| Distilled vinegar | raw apple cider vinegar, unpasteurized vinegars, or lemon juice | adjust to taste |

| Hydrogenated fats, oils & shortening | extra virgin olive oil or expeller pressed oils | using liquid fats instead of solid fats requires less liquid in recipe |
|---|---|---|
| Chocolate | carob powder or organic chocolate | 3 Tbs. carob plus 2 Tbs. milk powder equals 1 oz. chocolate |
| Sugar | natural sweeteners, pure maple syrup, evaporated cane syrup, barley malt, agave, raw honey, rice syrup, date sugar | Requires more dry ingredients or less liquid in recipe |
| Sodas | natural fruit juice, natural flavored sodas, sparkling water | |
| Coffee/Tea | Green or white tea, organic coffee, or herbal teas | Try it iced! |
| Canned or frozen vegetables | Fresh and organic fruits and vegetables | At least 40% higher in nutrients |

| High fat salad dressings | There are many good salad dressing on the market – avoid corn syrup, hydrogenated fats and artificial preservatives | Or make your own – see *Fresh Garden Salads* chapter in *The Passionate Vegetable* |
|---|---|---|
| Red meats and poultry | Natural beef, free range or organic chicken or vegetable protein—beans, tofu, nuts or seeds | |
| Pasta—white flour | Whole grain pastas, wheat free pastas or organic flour pastas | Needs to cook a little longer. Follow pkg. directions |
| Eggs | Organic and free-range eggs | You can taste the difference! |
| White Bread | Whole grain breads or whole grain sprouted breads | Better nutrients and fiber. Will satisfy you with less. |
| Whole milk and dairy | Organic dairy or dairy substitutes— rice milk, coconut, almond, or nut milks | Please read *Not Milk?* in Chapter 1 |
| Hydrogenated Margarine | Earth Balance organic buttery spread | |

# Chapter 5

## Pantry and Equipment Essentials and Techniques

## Pantry Essentials

My pantry is well stocked with a wide variety of ingredients so I always have on hand what I need when my creative culinary urge hits. It is certainly not necessary to have every one of these ingredients in your kitchen! I am so well stocked I could whip up something for several unexpected guests at a moment's notice.

**Condiments:** sea salt, oils, soy sauce, vinegars, miso, organic mayonnaise, mustard and ketchup to name a few. I have quite a large selection of dried herbs and spices. Most cooks can get by with twelve or so essential herbs and spices. I prefer mixing my own, so I purchase single herbs from the bulk section of a health food store as they are fresher and cheaper. Then I refill the empty store-bought jars or label my own.

**Sea Salt**: Use only natural sea salt. Natural sea salt contains trace elements and minerals. You will find that you may need less in a recipe. Read more in *Salt of the Earth* in Chapter 1.

**Oils:** I keep a variety of oils in my pantry, including extra virgin olive oil (for almost everything except frying); light sesame oil for pan frying and some salad dressings when I don't want an olive flavor; toasted sesame oil for Asian dishes; hot chili oil for a touch of heat in just about anything; and corn oil for baked goods. Unrefined corn oil is thick and rich like melted butter. Every oil imparts a unique flavor and consistency, and some recipes do better with one over the other.

> *Look for unrefined expeller pressed oils found in health food stores.*

If a recipe calls for a solid fat like butter, margarine or shortening and you want to substitute with oil, you must compensate for the liquid. Either add a tablespoon or two of flour to bring it up to its original consistency or reduce the oil. Oil is 100% fat, and butter is a combination of fat, water and whey, so don't use the same measurement or it will be too oily. If a recipe calls for ½ cup of butter, use 1/3 cup of oil to achieve the same richness. There are also "prunes pureed with flaxseed butters" available that are meant to be used instead of oil or eggs. Spectrum Naturals makes a vegetable shortening that is non-hydrogenated and can be found in health food stores. A non-hydrogenated margarine free of trans fats is Earth Balance. Again, it is found in health food stores.

*The quality of oils you use in your cooking will greatly affect the flavor of your dish!*

**Soy Sauce or Tamari**—Traditionally, tamari was the name given to soy sauce that was aged without wheat. That's no longer the case today. Soy sauce and tamari are essentially the same except that tamari tends to have a less salty taste. Be sure to get authentic soy sauce, without artificial ingredients and preservatives. If you are allergic to wheat, do read the labels.

**Vinegars**—I keep a variety of vinegars in my kitchen. My favorite brand is Spectrum Natural vinegars because they are unpasteurized. Similar in health value to the bacteria in yogurt, unpasteurized vinegars continue to ferment and age in the bottle. If you purchase one of these vinegars you may want to keep them refrigerated. If they get cloudy, that is a good sign and you should continue to use it in your recipes. There are many varieties available. Braggs Apple Cider Vinegar is the best and perhaps the only raw unpasteurized apple cider vinegar available. White distilled vinegar is too acidic and too processed to be used for food but is great for cleaning carpet stains! Occasionally, I'll purchase or make herb or fruit infused specialty vinegars.

**Herbs and Spices**—I stock a wide variety of dried herbs and spices and I also keep some fresh ones on hand. To keep them fresh, place fresh herbs such as parsley, dill and cilantro in a glass jar, with a few inches of water, and cover with a plastic bag. Keep refrigerated up to 10 days and change water every few days. For more information read *Cooking with Herbs and Spices.*

**Whole Grains**—These are the staple carbohydrates in our house, replacing the pasta and breads of my childhood diet. Although we still enjoy whole grain breads or pasta, it is not our daily fare. I keep a variety of rice on hand that includes brown basmati, short grain brown rice, and wild rice. I always stock millet, quinoa, barley and whole oats. You can include bulgur wheat, couscous and buckwheat too. If you are new to cooking whole grains, there are some mixes available on the market.

**Baking Ingredients**—I keep a typical selection of baking ingredients in my pantry except that all my ingredients are organic and whole-grain based. You will find unbleached flour, whole wheat flour and aluminum-free baking powder among my vanilla extract, spices and natural sweeteners.

**Pasta**—The pastas I frequently use in my recipes are whole grain pastas, rice noodles for Thai cooking, udon, somen, or soba (buckwheat pasta) for Asian dishes. Whole grain pastas will have more fiber and protein than conventional white pastas but not as much as the whole grain itself. Look for whole grain pastas with at least seven grams of protein and six grams of fiber per serving. It is a light, easy to digest occasional meal. I serve pasta once a week during hot weather.

**Beans**—Keep a variety of dried beans and some canned beans on hand such as adzuki, black beans, great northern, navy, pinto, garbanzo (chickpeas), red or green lentils, as well as split green peas. I always prepare more than I need and freeze the remainder in dinner size portions for later use. See my *Bean Cuisine* chapter in *The Passionate Vegetable* cookbook for helpful hints on how to successfully cook beans.

**Extras in a Can**—Some extras that come in handy and can be kept in your pantry are a variety of canned organic tomatoes, capers, sun-dried tomatoes, olives and light coconut milk. These ingredients sometimes show up in my recipes, so they are always good to keep on hand. I also stock organic frozen corn and peas year round in the freezer.

**Extras**—Additional pantry items would include hot and cold cereals and non-dairy milks.

**Sweeteners**—For flavor and nutrition, I prefer using pure maple syrup, as well as raw honey, brown rice syrup, barley malt or agave syrup. In a recipe, if you are exchanging a dry ingredient (white or brown sugar) for a wet one, you can use the same amount but add a little flour to the recipe to bring it back to its original consistency. See *The Real Scoop on Sugar* in Chapter 1.

**Sea Vegetables**—Not your common "beach seaweed," sea vegetables are cultivated and harvested specifically for food consumption. They have been a major part of Asian diets and coastal cultures since ancient times. Very alkalizing and full of minerals, you will find sea vegetables quite flavorful. Hiziki, for instance, contains fourteen times more calcium than a glass of milk! I keep kombu, wakame flakes, dulse, nori, hiziki, and arame in my pantry. My kids and I love them all!

**Nuts and Seeds**—Using nuts and seeds in whole grain dishes adds protein, good quality fat and makes for a surprising texture. I always stock almonds, walnuts, peanuts, pecans and pine nuts as I never know when the urge to snack or throw a handful in a recipe might stir me. Keep them in the refrigerator or freezer to extend their freshness.

**Dried Fruit**—Use organic or sulfur-free dried fruits whenever possible. Most conventionally grown produce will have pesticide residuals and drying the fruit only concentrates these chemicals. Mostly for baking, I keep organic dried cranberries, raisins, currants, figs, apricots and apples in my refrigerator. Sometimes they find their way into salads or into whole grain dishes. My kids like to snack on them as well. They are a nutritious sweet alternative.

**Onions and Garlic**—These are staples in my house because I'm not sure I would know how to cook without them! Check my blog www.suzannelandry.com for helpful video tutorials on how to chop an onion without crying.

# Equipment Essentials

Although I don't believe it is necessary to buy special equipment for natural foods cooking, there are some tools that I find essential for whatever cooking I am doing.

**Stove:** I mention this because I believe strongly that healthy food cannot be prepared on electric stoves. Food tastes better and is better cooked with natural gas. Gas flames are easier to control. Electric burners are harder to control and can easily overcook or dry out food.

**Cookware:** All metal weakens with repeated heating and cooling, which expands and contracts the metal, allowing leaching of the metal into our food. Though it will take a few years, even stainless steel will leach eventually. Most health-oriented professional chefs use heavy clad stainless steel, cast iron, or baked enamel cookware. Aluminum, a weaker metal, leaches quickly into our food and is absorbed into our bodies. Please replace aluminum cookware as soon as you can. Nonstick cookware also leaches even when it hasn't been scratched. You can purchase nonstick cookware that is non-toxic. Look for "green pans" or eco cookware in your local kitchen department store.

**Cutting Boards:** Yes, wood is best! Acrylic boards dull knives quickly. Further, bacteria lives on wet surfaces and moisture stays on acrylic boards longer; whereas wooden boards absorb the moisture. However, I do recommend acrylic boards for meat and chicken. You may want sterilize them in the dishwasher after each use. Some cooks like to have a separate small board for onion and garlic chopping. I use a wooden board that is at least one to two-inches thick and pieced together. A solid piece of wood will warp. A board 12 x 14 inches is a good size. You can ask at a wood furniture store or hobby shop if they will custom make your board from scrap wood or you can purchase one at a good kitchen shop.

Monthly, I sterilize my boards by wiping the surface with a solution of 50% water and 50% vinegar. The following day I oil the surface thoroughly with light cooking oil. My boards have lasted for many years and don't show signs of wear. By the way, never put a wooden board in the dishwasher or wash it in soapy water or with a soapy sponge. If you use a wood board for vegetables and fruits, wipe it down with a hot sponge without soap. I have a designated cutting board sponge that never gets used for washing dishes or for general cleanup. Your board will last for many years when you take proper care of it.

**Egg Slicer:** It can multi-task beyond boiled eggs. Use it for slicing hulled strawberries or firm mushrooms.

**Essentials:** Small essentials can include measuring cups, garlic press, spatulas, citrus juicer, storage containers, a variety of small kitchen knives and of course, your favorite gadgets.

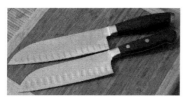

**Knives**: If you want to cut vegetables with ease and speed, invest in a good knife and keep it sharp. You don't have to spend a lot of money on a knife but there are some features to look for. One of my favorite, yet inexpensive knives is a Santoku style from Cuisinart. Stainless steel is easier to clean but doesn't stay sharp as long as carbon steel. Ceramic blades stay sharp much longer, but are brittle when dropped. Additionally, a couple of very good paring knives are all you'll need. Knife sharpening can be done with a whet stone, steel rod or an electric sharpener, whichever you are most comfortable with. Note: you can sustain a more serious cut injury with a dull knife than with a sharp one. Sharpen your knives once a week. Invest in a good knife, buy it at a kitchenware shop and ask them to give you a demonstration on knife sharpening.

**Food Processor**: Every kitchen should have a food processor because it can be used for blending soups, chopping nuts and vegetables and mixing just about everything. You don't need an expensive processor with many attachments. Most of those extra gadgets you won't use anyway. The high-powered blenders available are great for vegetable and fruit smoothies and protein breakfast drinks.

**Ginger Grater:** This is an easy and inexpensive tool if you frequently use fresh ginger as I do. A small handheld cheese grater can also work.

**Juicer:** If you are serious about stepping up your health and vitality a notch or more, then a juicer is a necessity. For those who work, it is nearly impossible to get the five servings of fruits and vegetables in our daily diet. The easiest way to sneak in more of these veggies and fruit and the antioxidant protection they bring, is to juice. I will bring 16 ounces of fresh squeezed vegetable and fruit juice with me most workdays. I can see a difference in my skin when I do that. It looks smoother and softer and more youthful. The juicer I have now is a Green Star. It is a low speed twin gear juicer that gently crushes and squeezes my veggies so they don't heat up, which destroys nutrients, antioxidants, and enzymes. I prefer this style of juicer to the basket type that shreds and spins the produce at high speed. This high speed will begin to oxidize the enzymes in the juice and because of that you should drink the juice within 15 minutes. It's faster than mine but the pulp comes out wetter and you get less juice for your money with these styles.

**Immersion Blender:** Also known as a handheld blender. I love this tool! These blenders are designed to blend soup, gravies, and sauces without removing them from pot. It saves time and mess. They are available in most kitchen department stores. Hold it down in your pot of soup and blend away without dirtying any other equipment!

**Microwave:** I don't use it . . . not even for heating foods. There are other methods of reheating and cooking food that are far more healthful.

**Pressure Cooker:** While not an essential piece of equipment, a pressure cooker does cut cooking time in half when cooking beans. Rice tastes sweeter when cooked in a pressure cooker. Use only stainless steel or enamel, not an aluminum pressure cooker. Aluminum, as mentioned before, will leach easier into food than stainless steel.

**Salad Spinner:** I use mine everyday. Easy to wash, drain and spin your salad. You can even store it in the bowl. I like the Zyliss style because it is easy to use and nearly indestructible.

**Scissors:** Get kitchen shears meant for cutting chicken bones and skin. Scissors are an invaluable tool to keep in the kitchen for snipping herbs, cutting up dried fruit or whole tomatoes in a can, and trimming fat from meats.

**Toaster Oven:** This is another frequently used item in my kitchen. I use it for toasting nuts or seeds, melting cheese on tortillas, and reheating food. It saves energy and time. Why heat a whole oven (and the whole house) to cook one small dish?

**Vegetable Peeler:** Unless a vegetable has been waxed, I recommend not peeling it. The most versatile peeler is the one that looks like a sling shot. The blade is placed horizontally and you simply pull the peeler along the surface of the vegetable. It saves your knuckles and is the best tool for hard-to-peel vegetables like squash. It is one of my most frequently used tools. My favorite is the Kuhn from Sweden.

**Water Ionizer:** Drinking ionized, clustered (restructured) water everyday can improve your health and overall well being. We chose the Kangen Water Ionizer because of its quality and versatility. This machine gives me a wide range of pH choices for water not only for drinking (from 7 pH to 9.5 pH alkaline) but for disinfecting everything from my countertops to my chopping blocks as well. Most importantly, this 2.5 pH is acidic enough to kill most salmonella, E. coli and other pathogens within 30 seconds. I soak my vegetables in this water for 30 seconds and then put them in an alkaline water of 11.5 pH. This pH will help to remove pesticide residue from all my produce (even organic vegetables get rained on). Meats and chicken will also get a quick 30-second bath in the 2.5 pH water. My fresh food is squeaky clean by the time I'm ready to prepare it. We use 8.5 pH to cook with and drink and love the flavor.

For information go to chapter 2, *Healthiest Water for Cooking and Drinking* or online www.LivingWaterforLife.com.

# Cooking Techniques

Every cook has her/his own special way of doing things, so I'll define my favorite cooking methods. Remember: cooking destroys most enzymes, so be sure that you include raw vegetables and fruit everyday. This insures that you will get a well balanced diet that includes enzymes, vitamins and minerals.

**Steaming**—Most vegetables are best when steamed as steaming retains moisture, flavor and nutrients. In steaming, the water should never touch the vegetables and should boil gently. A handy tool for steaming is an expandable steamer basket which adjusts to fit different size pots. You can buy one just about anywhere these days. It takes only a little bit longer to steam on the stove than to microwave with better nutrient retention.

**Blanching**—This is a very quick way to cook vegetables. This is the method used prior to freezing vegetables. The water remains boiling while vegetables are placed in the water for a very brief period of time. The vegetable is then immediately plunged into iced cold water for several seconds to stop the cooking and then drained. Vegetables should be brightly colored and still have a fresh crisp taste without sacrificing nutrients. I use this method for some vegetables that will go in salads but are difficult to digest raw such as broccoli and cauliflower. I've blanched the vegetables that will go in my *Cauliflower and String Bean Dijon Salad* recipe in the *Fresh Garden Salads* chapter in my cookbook, *The Passionate Vegetable*.

**Boiling**—This technique is most often used for whole grains, beans, soups, stews and some vegetables. First the water is brought to a high boil, vegetables are added and then the temperature is lowered to a low boil for the remaining cooking time. Cover the pot to prevent evaporation and to have better control over cooking time.

**Sauté**—This method of cooking uses low heat and a small amount of oil. Sautéing is usually used for vegetables that have high moisture content, like onions and mushrooms.

**Stir-Fry**—Stir-fried vegetables are crispier and tastier than boiled or steamed. In this method of cooking, high heat and oil is used to quickly sear vegetables. Add vegetables according to their cooking time. Usually a small quantity of water or stock is added, the pot is covered and the vegetables cook in the steam. See my *Vegetable Stir-Fry with Teriyaki Sauce* in my *Vegetables—Nature's Bounty* chapter in my cookbook, *The Passionate Vegetable*.

**Baking**—Is an alternative way to cook grains, meats, beans, and vegetables. Sweet vegetables such as onions, carrots, squash, and parsnips become sweeter when they are baked. Always preheat your oven for 15 minutes before baking to ensure even heat and consistent cooking time. Vegetables can also be wrapped in foil and then baked or grilled.

**Roasting**—Usually cooked in a hot oven over 400 degrees. It carmelizes the sweetness out of root vegetables. See *Roasted Winter Vegetables* in *Vegetables–Nature's Bounty* in *The Passionate Vegetable*.

**Pressure Cooking**—A pressure cooker can reduce the cooking time of beans by almost half. However, lentils, black-eye peas, soybeans, and split peas should never be cooked in a pressure cooker. The foam that is created when cooking these beans will clog the vent of the pressure cooker. Also, be careful to not overfill a pressure cooker; filling to two thirds of capacity to allow for expansion of beans and grains. Grains cooked this way retain their flavor better too. I prefer the taste of pressure cooked rice over boiled.

**Deep Frying**—This method of cooking is very high in fat calories, so use it moderately. If you deep fry, be sure to use an oil that does not smoke at high temperatures. Good options for high heat are peanut, canola or sunflower oils. It is very important to make sure oil is hot enough before adding food. Food placed in oil should begin to sizzle immediately. If it does not, the oil is not hot enough and the food will absorb an excessive amount of oil, making the food soggy. Also, do not crowd the pan with too much food. The more food, the quicker the oil temperature will cool and the soggier the dish will be. Fill only half the surface of the pan with food to be fried.

**Reheating Food**: Avoid using the microwave so you can retain more nutrients. If you enjoyed a great meal, and want to reheat leftovers another day, you can make a plate of food and put the plate inside a bamboo steamer basket, cover and set it inside a skillet of water and bring water to boil. Foods will steam-heat in 5 minutes and you only have one plate to wash. Bamboo steamer baskets are inexpensive and can be found in Asian food markets or kitchen specialty stores. You can also reheat leftovers in an inexpensive stainless steel steamer basket placed inside a covered pot. Or wrap the plate in aluminum foil and place in a preheated 325°F toaster oven for 15 minutes. Careful, the plate will be hot!

# Measurements

I use standard American measuring cups. You can use the same measuring cup for both wet and dry ingredients. The weight differs from dry to weight ingredients but not the volume. For your information, I never refer to weight in my recipes.

Measurement by Cups: Liquid Ounces

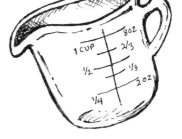

    1 cup = (8 oz)
    2 cups = 1 pint (16 oz)
    2 pints = 1 quart (32 oz)
    4 quarts = 1 gallon (64 oz)

**Measuring Spoons**—Use whatever spoons or measuring gadget you have that indicates fractions of teaspoons or tablespoons. Oval deep spoons are better than round shallow spoons, as it is easier to scoop out the ingredients. My recipes will refer to tablespoon by using the abbreviation of *Tbs.* and teaspoons as *tsp.* I believe most cooking measurements are standard and well understood with the possible exception of the pinch/dash (see below).

**Pinch/Dash**—This usually refers to salt or pepper. A pinch is the very smallest amount that you can pick up between two fingers; you probably could count the grains of salt. Dash is as much as you can quickly pick up between two fingers or one quick shake from the container.

# Knife Skills

All vegetables should be washed or scrubbed thoroughly before cutting. You should cut vegetables appropriate for the method of cooking you will be doing. For example, if you are creating a winter casserole of root vegetables which includes carrots, and it will cook for 30 minutes, cut carrots in large stew-sized pieces. On the other hand, if you are stir-frying carrots, cut them into thin diagonal slices or matchsticks so they cook quickly.

When cutting vegetables, it is easiest to use a knife with a rectangular cutting blade. Hold the knife by the handle close to the blade, with your thumb firmly placed on the side of the handle. You should feel you have a very good grip on the knife blade. Hold the vegetable with your other hand, with your fingers tucked under, using your knuckles to guide the vegetable toward the knife. The hand holding the vegetable should be cupped as if you were holding an egg in the palm of your hand.

The front end of the knife should remain on the board in front of the vegetable you are cutting. As you lift the back end of the blade just high enough over the vegetables to slice it, move the vegetable toward the knife while you continue to raise the back end of the knife and slice again, creating a rocking action. For a short demonstration video go to You Tube and look for *The Passionate Vegetable* or go to my blog www.suzannelandry.com.

The following cuts are most frequently used:

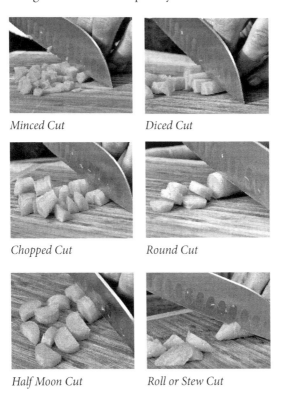

*Minced Cut*          *Diced Cut*

*Chopped Cut*         *Round Cut*

*Half Moon Cut*       *Roll or Stew Cut*

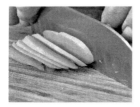
*Diagonal Cut*

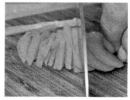
*Small Matchstick*

**Minced**—about ¼ of an inch cube

**Diced**—about ⅓ of an inch cube

**Chopped**—about ½ of an inch cube

**Rounds**—cut across a round vegetable such as a carrot

**Half Moon Cut**—slice in half lengthwise once and then crosswise in desired width

**Roll/Stew Cut**—very thick diagonal cut—roll vegetable toward you and cut through the flat facing of the vegetable and diagonally cut again. Keep rolling and cutting across diagonally. You should end up with triangular-shaped vegetables.

**Diagonal**—cut a vegetable at an angle (on the diagonal)

**Matchstick**—cut diagonally, then into thin strips about 1 inch long

**Quarter Cut**—As in a tomato or onion. Cut in half and half again ending up with four quarters.

## Other books by Suzanne Landry:

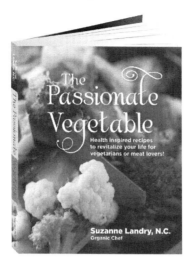

More than 300 pages of easy and delicious recipes throughout nine chapters, scrumptious photographs and inspiring health information. Dramatically improve your health and energy with mouthwatering recipes that can help you:

- *restore your youthful vitality*
- *end your cravings and feel more nourished*
- *satisfy your nutrition needs whether you are a vegetarian, flexitarian or meat lover*

More than a cookbook, it reveals the pure simplicity and bountiful flavor of fresh vegetables with recipes that range from earthy to elegant using simple everyday ingredients. You will also find a simple guide to food nutrition: pantry makeovers, 145 time-savers to make cooking fun again, discovering fresh herbs and spices, navigating the carbohydrate maze and suggestions for delicious vegetarian meals and much more.

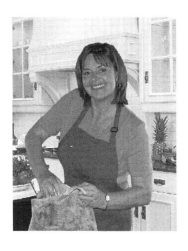

Ready to start cooking with

# Fresh Food?

Suzanne Landry's

*The Passionate Vegetable*

is now available at

www.ThePassionateVegetable.com

and to help get you started I'll give you a 10% discount on The Passionate Vegetable! Just write to me at info@thepassionatevegetable.com and mention the code "PVDiscount"!

# Other Inspired Living Titles

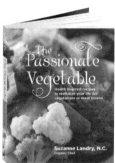

www.ThePassionateVegetable.com

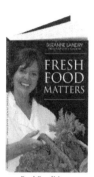

www.FreshFoodMatters.com

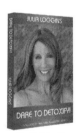

www.DareToDetoxify.com

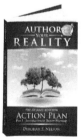

www.AuthorYourDreams.com

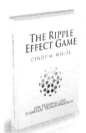

www.RippleEffectGame.com

# Health Inspired Publishing

We publish books that inspire healthy lifestyles.

For information, inspirational blogs and recipes visit
*www.suzannelandry.com.*

Suzanne is available for:

–   private cooking instruction
–   group cooking classes
–   speaking engagements
–   wellness consultations

If you would like information regarding this book, cooking classes, newsletters, and/or future publications, please let us know by giving us your contact information or write to us at *info@thepassionatevegetable.com.*

*Praise for The Passionate Vegetable*

"We just received the copy of *The Passionate Vegetable*. WOW! What an achievement. Superior production values. Excellent presentation. We had just purchased two other cookbooks recently (*Better Homes New Cookbook* 15th edition and *Moosewood Restaurant Cooking for Health*) but clearly yours outclasses them both with the text and the great illustrations. Thanks, it's impressive." –Jeffrey & Shayne T., Vermont

"WOW, you did an amazing job, the book is so beautiful, and way bigger and more beautiful than I expected. Can't wait to start cooking!" –Shirley D., Texas

"I just received my book. Big congratulations are in order – it is quite an achievement. It is such an impressive book and the photos look so bright and vibrant – it's beautiful." –Celia F., New York

"I received my new cookbook, *The Passionate Vegetable* and am really thrilled. It was kind of a coincidence that when it arrived, I was making your Lentil and Wild Rice Salad recipe, from a SBCC class that my husband and I took a couple of years ago. Thanks for completing the book, my family, friends, and I look forward to enjoying many of your tasty and nutritious recipes. Not to mention, all of your Bites of Insight." –Denise B., Washington

"For over a year we have eagerly awaited the publication of your book. The organization, layout, and descriptions of the recipes are perfect. It was worth the wait. Tonight I tried *Blackened Red*

*Snapper with Corn Relish*, which turned out as advertised. The spicy snapper against the "cool" relish was perfect. I anticipate enjoying many more of your recipes." –Bob B., North Carolina

"LOOKS FANTASTIC! BRAVO! What an awesome achievement! I will treasure it, and can't wait to try out the recipes." –Samantha B., California

"I received your book and it is beautiful!!! The photographs are stunning and the huge number of fantastic sounding recipes is so impressive. I love your "Bites of Insights" too. So, congratulations on a stunning achievement. I will include it in our next Edible Books column in *Edible Santa Barbara* magazine."–Krista H., California

Made in the USA
San Bernardino, CA
26 April 2014